S. HRG. 115–48

NATIVE YOUTH: PROMOTING DIABETES PREVENTION THROUGH HEALTHY LIVING

HEARING

BEFORE THE

COMMITTEE ON INDIAN AFFAIRS
UNITED STATES SENATE

ONE HUNDRED FIFTEENTH CONGRESS

FIRST SESSION

MARCH 29, 2017

Printed for the use of the Committee on Indian Affairs

U.S. GOVERNMENT PUBLISHING OFFICE

26–197 PDF   WASHINGTON : 2017

For sale by the Superintendent of Documents, U.S. Government Publishing Office
Internet: bookstore.gpo.gov   Phone: toll free (866) 512–1800; DC area (202) 512–1800
Fax: (202) 512–2104   Mail: Stop IDCC, Washington, DC 20402–0001

CONTENTS

NATIVE YOUTH: PROMOTING DIABETES PREVENTION THROUGH HEALTHY LIVING

WEDNESDAY, MARCH 29, 2017

U.S. SENATE,
COMMITTEE ON INDIAN AFFAIRS,
Washington, DC.

The Committee met, pursuant to notice, at 2:45 p.m. in room 628, Dirksen Senate Office Building, Hon. John Hoeven, Chairman of the Committee, presiding.

OPENING STATEMENT OF HON. JOHN HOEVEN, U.S. SENATOR FROM NORTH DAKOTA

The CHAIRMAN. Good afternoon. We will call this hearing to order.

Up front, I want to thank all our panelists for being here.

Today the Committee will hold an oversight hearing on Native Youth: Promoting Diabetes Prevention through Healthy Living.

In 1997, Congress authorized the Special Diabetes Program for Indians to address the extraordinary prevalence of diabetes among Indians. It is now in its twentieth year and up for reauthorization this year.

This program has demonstrated significant inroads in reducing diabetes and its complications, such as limb amputations, heart disease and kidney failure. However, there is still more work to be done.

Indian people have a greater chance of being diagnosed with diabetes than any other racial or ethnic group in the Country. It is the fifth leading cause of death for Native people. This disease is now afflicting the youth.

Native youth are reportedly nine times higher than non-Hispanic whites to be diagnosed with Type 2 diabetes and the related complications of heart disease, kidney failure, and other diseases.

I look forward to hearing from our witnesses regarding why, according to Indian Health Service information, and during the existence of this special program, the rates of diabetes among the youth have increased and obesity rates have pretty much stayed the same.

As we know, obesity is one indicator for the future risk of becoming diabetic. If it is not decreasing, then before we reauthorize this program and talk about a funding authorization level, we need to examine how well this special program is serving the Native American youth.

We know, on the bright side, Type 2 diabetes is both preventable and manageable, particularly through healthy living. Healthier lifestyles can help improve blood glucose levels, decrease obesity rates, lower blood pressure, and decrease bad cholesterol levels for our youth.

Today we look forward to hearing from our witnesses on how they are making a difference in the lives of Native youth and any improvements needed for this special program. We must work together to prevent further diabetes prevalence in Indian Country and continue the good work that is currently being done.

With that, I want to start with a special welcome to one of our witnesses today. Again, I welcome all of you but a special welcome to a witness from my home State of North Dakota, Mr. Jared Eagle. Thank you for being here from the Three Affiliated Tribes in New Town, North Dakota.

I want to thank all of you for being here and welcome you.

I also want to turn to Vice Chairman Udall for any opening statement he would like to make.

STATEMENT OF HON. TOM UDALL,
U.S. SENATOR FROM NEW MEXICO

Senator UDALL. Thank you very much, Chairman Hoeven, for calling this oversight hearing on Native Youth and Diabetes Prevention.

Too often in this Committee, we hear about the challenges facing Indian Country but I hope today's hearing will give us an opportunity to focus on the success stories. Throughout my time in public service, I have been fortunate to get to know some truly inspiring Native youth. Whether it is meeting with students from the Santa Fe Indian School on a trip to D.C. or joining kids from Santa Clara Pueblo's Youth Running Club for a run back in New Mexico, the one thing I always hear when I talk with Native youth is how important community, culture and mentorship are to their success.

As a committee, we should look for more ways to support the efforts of tribes and Native communities to engage Native youth in healthy lifestyles. I am glad we are here to learn more about the positive impact that culturally informed community health promotion programs can have in Indian Country.

One of the main ways Congress has supported tribally-driven diabetes prevention initiatives over the last 20 years has been through authorizing the Special Diabetes Program for Indians, otherwise known by the acronym SDPI. SDPI funds diabetes prevention and treatment programs in more than 300 Native communities across the Country, resulting in a 61 percent increase in culturally-based diabetes education programs.

The SDPI impact can be measured by more than statistics and health care cost savings. This program has helped to improve the quality of life for thousands of diabetic and pre-diabetic American Indians and Alaska Natives. I am sure many of the witnesses here today can attest to the positive impacts SDPI has had on their communities.

Despite the outstanding impact this program has had over the last two decades, it has suffered under the strain of one to two year reauthorizations. These short-term extensions have made it difficult for tribal diabetes programs to plan for the long term.

That is why I introduced a bill to reauthorize SDPI for another seven years. This long-term extension will provide Native grantees with peace of mind during the annual appropriations process and it makes a commonsense investment in preventive health care programs that will curb ever increasing medical costs.

I will conclude by inviting other members of this Committee in support of reauthorization of SDPI. I look forward to hearing from our witnesses about the innovative work SDPI has helped fund in their communities.

Thank you again, Mr. Chairman, for focusing on diabetes and prevention in this Committee.

The CHAIRMAN. Thank you, Senator Udall.

Are there other members who would like to make an opening statement?

STATEMENT OF HON. STEVE DAINES, U.S. SENATOR FROM MONTANA

Senator DAINES. Thank you, Chairman Hoeven and Vice Chairman Udall.

Let me tell you a story. It is the story of Dustin Mitchell.

Dustin is 14 years old. He is a member of the Confederated Salish and Kootenai Tribes of the Flathead Reservation in Northwest Montana. He is a regular, fun loving kid. He plays football, goes to school, and drives race car competition in the summer.

In 2012, he was diagnosed with diabetes. The diagnosis came as a shock to him and his family. The Mitchells did not have other family members who had struggled with diabetes before and needed to learn how to cope with Dustin's new challenge.

Soon thereafter, Dustin attended the American Diabetes Association's Camp Montana in Fishtail, Montana. There is a name for you, Fishtail, Montana, a beautiful place in our State. That is where he went to camp. He learned about healthy eating, exercise and how to manage his diabetes.

Now, Dustin still plays football in the summer and he is still racing racecars but this year, his Bandolero race car will feature a large sticker that will read "Hope," along with the signature diabetes awareness blood drop that calls attention of others to this epidemic.

Native children ages 10 to 19 years old are nine times more likely than their young Caucasian counterparts to be diagnosed with Type 2 diabetes. Through lifestyle adaptations like the ones Dustin made and by supporting the Special Diabetes for Indians Program, which every Montana tribe benefits from, we can prevent more Indian children and adults alike from becoming diabetic.

Thank you, Mr. Chairman.

The CHAIRMAN. Thank you, Senator Daines.

Senator Franken.

STATEMENT OF HON. AL FRANKEN,
U.S. SENATOR FROM MINNESOTA

Senator FRANKEN. Thank you, Chairman Hoeven and Vice Chairman Udall, for calling this oversight hearing.

Thank you to all of our witnesses for your testimony today. I look forward to hearing your testimony. I will keep my remarks very brief.

Many of us in this room have spent years working on this issue. For me, diabetes was the topic of the second Floor speech I gave when I became a U.S. Senator. It has been an issue I have worked on ever since. We are all aware of the toll of diabetes on families across the Nation, specifically of course in Indian Country which is why this hearing is an important opportunity for this Committee to take up this important issue, one that is so prevalent among our Indian youth.

Thank you again, Mr. Chairman and Ranking Member, and all of our witnesses. I look forward to your testimony.

The CHAIRMAN. Senator Cortez Masto.

STATEMENT OF HON. CATHERINE CORTEZ MASTO,
U.S. SENATOR FROM NEVADA

Senator CORTEZ MASTO. Chairman Hoeven, thank you so much and Ranking Member Udall.

This is a fantastic panel. I just wanted the opportunity, however, to introduce all of you to one of the panelists from the great State of Nevada. That is Chairman Vinton Hawley from the Lake Paiute Tribe located in Nevada. I am so pleased you were able to join us today.

Chairman Hawley is here today in his capacity as the Chair of the National Indian Health Board which represents tribal governments that both operate their own health care systems and those that rely on care provided through the Indian Health Service.

He also serves as President of the Nevada Intertribal Council, a network of 27 tribes and community organizations serving Indian people living in Nevada and the Great Basin region. He is a proud member of both the Pyramid Lake Paiute Tribe and the Hopi-Tewa. I am so happy he is here to join us today. Welcome to all of you and thank you.

The CHAIRMAN. Senator Murkowski.

STATEMENT OF HON. LISA MURKOWSKI,
U.S. SENATOR FROM ALASKA

Senator MURKOWSKI. Thank you, Mr. Chairman.

I too will be brief but I thank you for having this very important hearing today. I think we have recognized here in Congress that we are dealing with something that is epidemic in proportion and to know that we have dedicated funding through the SDPI program in hopes of obtaining better data, lowering the rates and making a real impact in the lives of not only children but all of Native Americans.

We have seen some encouraging signs in Alaska through the SDPI program as we deal with the diabetes epidemic today. We have 19 Native organizations or tribes participating in programs across the State.

We still have a pretty big problem. According to CDC, in 2014, approximately 41,181 in Alaska, 7.6 percent of the population had been diagnosed with diabetes. We understand what this leads to in terms of other serious conditions.

It is not only the individual that has diabetes, it is the toll on the families as well as they care for their loved ones, but also the fact that it is passed down through generations, sometimes through factors such as poor eating habits, and a lack of a healthy lifestyle. Those too are passed down.

In Alaska, we have some additional challenges. In remote areas, when you have an inability to get good, healthy foods in a grocery store, your fruits and vegetables, they just do not exist or if they do, they are too expensive, so many of our Alaska Natives rely on good subsistence food whether it is moose, caribou or fish.

Sometimes these foods are not available, so you have to rely on less healthy alternatives which are costly and contribute to further challenges. Also, you have long winters that make healthy outside activities somewhat limited.

We are making some good progress. I think that is important, particularly the progress with our young people.

I would like to recognize one of our panelists this afternoon and thank him for joining us today. Martin Sensmeier was raised in Yakutat, Alaska, a small community, less than 1,000 people, a beautiful community. Martin is Tlingit and Koyukon-Athabascan.

I want to thank you for traveling here today, Martin. It is a long haul. We know that. The last time I saw you in D.C., you had once again traveled all the way across the Country to spend just one day, just one day, with Native youth. That truly was your personal statement and commitment to the mission and the cause that you lead so ably and competently. You are a role model for so many.

I thank you for that and I thank you for being here and providing us with your comments today.

With that, Mr. Chairman, I thank you.

The CHAIRMAN. Thank you, Senator Murkowski.

We are very pleased to have our witnesses today. They are: Rear Admiral Chris Buchanan, Acting Director, Indian Health Service, U.S. Department of Health and Human Services, Rockville, Maryland; The Honorable Vinton Hawley, Chair, National Indian Health Board, Washington, D.C.; Mr. Jared Eagle, Program Director, Fort Berthold Diabetes Program—Three Affiliated Tribes, New Town, North Dakota; Mr. Martin Sensmeier, Actor and Ambassador, Boys & Girls Clubs of America, Atlanta, Georgia, most recently in the movie The Magnificent Seven. We will get a few more details on his acting as well as diabetes. I know I am not the only one interested to hear a little bit more about that.

Mr. Alton Villegas is also here. He represents Tribal Youth from the Salt River Pima-Maricopa Indian Community, Scottsdale, Arizona. I understand they tried to take you out for a hamburger last night and you ordered a salad. Way to go. You are setting a good example right there. Ms. Rachel Seepie, Senior Fitness Specialist, Diabetes Service Program - Health Service, Salt River Pima-Maricopa Indian Community, Scottsdale, Arizona, is with him also.

Thanks again to all of you. If you will hold your comments to five minutes if you could, your full written statement will be made a part of the permanent record.

Admiral Buchanan.

STATEMENT OF REAR ADMIRAL CHRIS BUCHANAN, ACTING DIRECTOR, INDIAN HEALTH SERVICE, U.S. DEPARTMENT OF HEALTH AND HUMAN SERVICES

Mr. BUCHANAN. Good afternoon everyone. Good afternoon, Chairman Hoeven, Vice Chairman Udall, and members of the Committee.

My name is Chris Buchanan. I am an enrolled tribal member of the Seminole Nation of Oklahoma. I am a Commissioned Corps officer with the Public Health Service and the Acting IHS Director. I have been with the Indian Health Service for about 24 years and have held various levels of assignments within the Indian Health Service.

I am truly honored to be here to testify before the Senate Committee on Indian Affairs concerning Native youth and promoting diabetes prevention and healthy living.

Mr. Chairman, I want to thank you and Vice Chairman Udall for your leadership on the Committee and for elevating the importance of delivering quality health through the Indian Health Service.

Diabetes is a chronic disease, is complex and costly and requires tremendous long-term efforts to prevent and treat. American Indians and Alaska Native people are affected more by diabetes. Diabetes rates in these populations are more than twice that of non-Hispanic Whites in the United States.

I am happy to report after several decades of intensive efforts by the Indian Health programs and partners we are seeing clear evidence that this epidemic has leveled off. Within our communities, the years of increasing rates of diabetes stopped in 2011 and it has not risen since that time.

As shown by the graph to the left, new cases of kidney failure due to diabetes declined by 54 percent among American Indians and Alaska Native adults from 1996 to 2013. This is a much larger decline than in any other racial group in the United States.

As the future of Indian Country depends on the health of its youth, recent data shows there is good news here as well. The rate of Type 2 diabetes in American Indian youth ages 10 to 19 did not increase from 2001 to 2009.

Although the rate is still higher than other ethnic and racial groups, the rate of obesity in American Indian and Alaska Native youth has also leveled off. The obesity rate in American Indian and Alaska Native children ages 2 to 19 years remained nearly constant from 2006 to 2015. However, it is still higher than U.S. youth overall.

Several key factors contributed to this significant and ongoing progress including the Special Diabetes Program for Indians, also known as SDPI. Twenty years ago, in 1997, Congress created the SDPI in response to the diabetes epidemic that was escalating at an alarming rate in the Native population.

The SDPI Program provides grants to tribal IHS urban Indian Health organizations for diabetes prevention and treatment services. Grantees collectively serve over 782,000 American Indians and Alaska Native people per year. Two-thirds of the grantees use at least some of their SDPI funds to work with children and youth.

Examples of the services that grantees implement to reduce risk factors of obesity and diabetes in youth include school and community-based physical activity, nutrition and education, community gardens, American Indian and Alaska Native traditional sports and dancing and obesity management clinics.

In addition to the SDPI, the IHS has established partnerships to advance the health of Native youth and families. The Indian Health Service provides $1 million per year to support obesity prevention at Boys and Girls Clubs in Indian Country.

We do this through a cooperative agreement with the National Congress of American Indians. The NCAI awards funds to these clubs so that they can implement the program known as TRAIL. Over 14,000 Native youth have participated in the TRAIL program since 2003.

Although it takes many years to turn around an epidemic like diabetes, American Indians and Alaska Native communities are making a significant improvement in childhood obesity, diabetes prevalence and diabetes and kidney-related failure.

Thank you for your commitment to Native youth as well as your vision and leadership for diabetes prevention and treatment among American Indians and Alaska Native people.

I would be happy to answer any questions the Committee may have. Thank you.

[The prepared statement of Mr. Buchanan follows:]

PREPARED STATEMENT OF REAR ADMIRAL CHRIS BUCHANAN, ACTING DIRECTOR, INDIAN HEALTH SERVICE, U.S. DEPARTMENT OF HEALTH AND HUMAN SERVICES

Chairman and Members of the Committee:

Good afternoon, Chairman Hoeven, Vice-Chairman Udall, and Members of the Committee. I am Chris Buchanan, an enrolled member of the Seminole Nation of Oklahoma and currently the Acting Director of the Indian Health Service (IHS). Prior to that I was the IHS Deputy Director, leading and overseeing IHS operations to ensure delivery of quality comprehensive health services. I am pleased to have the opportunity to testify before the Senate Committee on Indian Affairs on our accomplishments in preventing diabetes for Native youth through our work in partnership with American Indian and Alaska Native (AI/AN) communities. I would like to thank you and Vice-Chairman Udall for your leadership on the Committee and for elevating the importance of delivering quality care through the Indian Health Service.

The IHS plays a unique role in the Department of Health and Human Services (HHS) because it is a health care system that was established to meet Federal trust responsibilities to American Indians and Alaska Natives. The mission of the IHS, in partnership with American Indian and Alaska Native people, is to raise the physical, mental, social, and spiritual health of AI/ANs to the highest level. The IHS provides comprehensive health service delivery to approximately 2.2 million AI/ANs through 26 hospitals, 59 health centers, 32 health stations, and nine school health centers. Tribes also provide healthcare access through an additional 19 hospitals, 284 health centers, 163 Alaska Village Clinics, 79 health stations, and eight school health centers.

Diabetes is a complex and costly chronic disease that requires tremendous long-term efforts to prevent and treat. Although diabetes is a nationwide public health problem, AI/AN people have been and remain disproportionately affected, with diabetes prevalence more than twice that for non-Hispanic whites in the United States. However, after several decades of intensive efforts by the IHS, Tribes, Urban Indian health organizations, and other partners, we are seeing clear evidence that this epidemic has leveled off.

In AI/AN people, the years of increasing diabetes prevalence stopped in 2011 and it has not risen since that time.[1] In addition, data show that focusing on quality, team-based clinical care has reduced devastating complications from diabetes. According to the January 2017 Centers for Disease Control and Prevention (CDC) Vital Signs report, new cases of diabetes-related kidney failure decreased dramatically (54 percent) among AI/AN adults from 1996 to 2013, a much larger decline than in any other racial group in the United States.[2] This decrease is especially important given that Medicare spent over $82,000 per person for beneficiaries of all races with diabetes-related, end-stage kidney disease in 2013.[3]

As the future of Indian Country depends on the health of its youth, recent data show that there is good news here as well. Although the prevalence of type 2 diabetes in American Indian (AI) youth ages 10–19 is higher than in other racial/ethnic groups, the prevalence for AI youth in this age group did not increase from 2001–2009. However, during that same period, it increased significantly for white, black, and Hispanic youth.[4] Even better, as it predicts future diabetes risk, the prevalence of obesity in AI/AN youth has also leveled off. Although higher than in US youth overall, obesity prevalence in AI/AN children and youth ages 2–19 years remained nearly constant from 2006–2015.[5] Several key factors contributed to this significant and ongoing progress, including the Special Diabetes Program for Indians (SDPI).

The SDPI was established by Congress in 1997 in response to the diabetes epidemic that was escalating at an alarming rate in AI/AN people. The SDPI provides grants to Tribal, IHS, and Urban Indian health organizations for diabetes prevention and treatment services. The IHS administers the SDPI grant program to promote evidence-based best practices as well as to ensure accountability for the funds and compliance with grants regulations. The SDPI 2014 Report to Congress documented the continued improvements in key clinical outcome measures since the inception of the SDPI. The SDPI is currently authorized at $150 million per year through the end of FY 2017.

Since the inception of SDPI, grantees have successfully implemented evidence-based and community-driven strategies to prevent and treat diabetes. There are currently 301 SDPI grant programs in 35 States, 252 Tribal, 20 IHS, and 29 Urban. Grantees collectively served over 782,000 AI/AN people per year, with two-thirds of grantees using at least some of their SDPI funding to work with children and youth. Examples of services that grantees implement to reduce risk factors for obesity and diabetes in youth include school and community-based physical activity and nutrition education, community gardens, AI/AN traditional sports and dancing, cooking classes, sports leagues, and obesity-management clinics. The innovative programs they have developed honor and incorporate their unique and diverse tribal cultures.

In addition to the SDPI, the IHS has established many partnerships to advance the health of Native youth and families. The IHS provides $1 million per year to support obesity prevention at Boys & Girls Clubs (Clubs) in Indian Country through a cooperative agreement with the National Congress of American Indians (NCAI). NCAI conducts an annual grant process to awards funds to Native Clubs so they can implement the Together Raising Awareness for Indian Life (TRAIL) program. TRAIL uses a comprehensive curriculum that includes educational, nutritional, and physical activities to promote healthy lifestyles, obesity prevention, and self-esteem for AI/AN youth. Over 14,000 AI/AN youth, ages seven through 11 years, have participated in the TRAIL program since 2003.

As important as it is to work with school-aged children, recent science has shown that risk factors for obesity and diabetes start in the earliest days and years of life. IHS has a Memorandum of Understanding with Johns Hopkins University's Center for American Indian Health to promote implementation of their evidence-based Family Spirit home visiting intervention. Working with pregnant women and young families, Family Spirit has been proven to reduce risk factors in American Indian

---

[1] IHS National Data Warehouse. 2016.

[2] Bullock A, Burrows NR, Narva AS, et al. Vital Signs: Decrease in Incidence of Diabetes-Related End-Stage Renal Disease among American Indians/Alaska Natives—United States, 1996–2013. MMWR Morb Mortal Wkly Rep 2017;66:26–32. DOI: http://dx.doi.org/10.15585/mmwr.mm6601e1.

[3] Id.

[4] Dabelea D, Mayer-Davis EJ, Saydah S, et al. Prevalence of Type 1 and Type 2 Diabetes Among Children and Adolescents From 2001 to 2009. JAMA 2014 May 7;311(17): 1778–1786.

[5] Ogden CL, Carroll MD, Lawman HG, et al. Trends in Obesity Prevalence Among Children and Adolescents in the United States, 1988–1994 Through 2013–2014. JAMA 2016:315 (21):2292–2299; IHS National Data Warehouse. 2016.

children that are associated with later development of obesity and substance abuse. [6]

Although it takes many years to turn around an epidemic like diabetes, this is happening in AI/AN communities, with significant improvements in childhood obesity, diabetes prevalence, and diabetes-related kidney failure. Thank you for your commitment to Native youth as well as your vision and leadership for diabetes prevention and treatment among AI/AN people. I look forward to continuing to work with you, our communities, and other partners to ensure the health of our Native youth and families. I will be happy to answer any questions the Committee may have.

The CHAIRMAN. Thank you, Admiral.
Mr. Hawley.

STATEMENT OF HON. VINTON HAWLEY, CHAIRPERSON, NATIONAL INDIAN HEALTH BOARD

Mr. HAWLEY. Chairman Hoeven, Vice Chairman Udall and members of the Committee, thank you for holding this important hearing on improving the lives and health of American Indian and Alaska Native youth through preventing diabetes.

My name is Vinton Hawley, Chairman of the Pyramid Lake Paiute Tribe, President of the Intertribal Council of Nevada and Chairperson of the National Indian Health Board. I appreciate the opportunity to provide this testimony today on behalf of the National Indian Health Board and the 567 Native Nations we serve.

One of the most prominent health disparities in tribal communities is the high rate of Type 2 diabetes. Our people of all ages are impacted by Type 2 diabetes and its many chronic complications whether through our own individual diagnosis or the diagnosis of a loved one.

Because of stories like this and the many tribal families who endure suffering because of Type 2 diabetes, tribal communities must have the resources and support they need to access fresh and nutritious foods, safe places for physical activity and quality diabetes treatment and intervention programs. Because traditional subsistence lifestyles have been replaced with Federal programs such as the Food Distribution Program on Indian reservations, many tribal communities have a new reliance on store-bought foods, poor access to fresh produce, and have increased consumption of fast foods.

These compounding issues have resulted in our children suffering from higher rates of obesity and related complications, such as Type 2 diabetes. Our Native youth ages 10–19 are nine times more likely to have Type 2 diabetes compared to non-Natives. This is unacceptable.

People with diabetes diagnosed before they turn 20 years old have a life expectancy that is up to 27 years shorter than people without diabetes.

One program in particular, the Special Diabetes Program for Indians, has been a major success for diabetes treatment and prevention programs throughout Indian Country. SDPI, as stated, was enacted by Congress in 1997. Along with its sister program for Type 1 diabetes research, it has become the Nation's most strategic, com-

---

[6] Barlow A, Mullany B, Neault N, et al. Paraprofessional-delivered, home-visiting intervention for American Indian teen mothers and children: 3-year outcomes from a randomized controlled trial. Am J Psychiatry 2015;172:154–162

prehensive and effective effort to combat diabetes and its complications.

This success is largely because communities design and implement their own diabetes interventions that are culturally appropriate. SDPI currently provides grants for over 300 programs in 35 States.

The success is shown in national data. Because of SDPI, our communities are reducing individual cholesterol levels, A1C levels and losing weight. Since SDPI started, end stage renal disease due to diabetes in our people has gone down by 54 percent.

Treatment for this is the biggest driver of Medicare costs, about $87,000 per patient per year just by reducing ESRD–D, we are saving the Federal Government millions of dollars a year and more importantly, saving the lives of our people.

SDPI is also improving entire tribal communities. For example, the Pyramid Lake Paiute Tribe focuses on diabetes education. Over the years, my tribe's diabetes education has evolved to be conveyed to our tribal youth that diabetes does not have to be a death sentence as it is often perceived.

Youth are also now more engaged with their aunts, uncles, grandmas and grandpas. They can help those family members know diabetes is manageable. We are living longer lives and SDPI is uniting communities, preserving cultures and filling generational gaps.

SDPI authorization is set to expire this September. We urge Congress to act swiftly to reauthorize SDPI and ensure continuity and the successful prevention and intervention efforts being conducted all across Indian Country. In addition to SDPI reauthorization, the National Indian Health Board has developed other recommendations for tribes and policymakers to pursue and strengthen diabetes prevention efforts for Native youth. In the interest of time, I would direct you to our written testimony for further detailed recommendations.

While tribes have made important gains in recent years in terms of Type 2 diabetes funding, improved health outcomes and the leveling off of diabetes incidence rates through initiatives like SDPI, there is still a long way to go before Native youth, children and families will no longer be devastated by the impacts of diabetes and its complications.

Thank you again for the opportunity to offer this statement. We appreciate being able to work together with you on this important issue. We look forward to working together on issues such as confirming an IHS director.

The National Indian Health Board and the 567 federally-recognized tribes we serve endorsed Dr. Charles Green as IHS director and will work with the Committee to achieve his confirmation.

Thank you. If you have any questions, I am more than happy to answer those.

[The prepared statement of Mr. Hawley follows:]

PREPARED STATEMENT OF VINTON HAWLEY, CHAIRPERSON, NATIONAL INDIAN HEALTH BOARD (NIHB)

Introduction

Chairman Hoeven, Vice Chairman Udall and Members of the Committee, thank you for holding this important hearing on improving the lives and health of American Indian and Alaska Native youth through preventing diabetes. Thank you for the opportunity to provide this testimony on behalf of the National Indian Health Board (NIHB).

The federal promise to provide for the health of Indian people was made long ago. Since the earliest days of the Republic, all branches of the federal government have acknowledged the nation's obligations to the Tribes and the special trust relationship between the United States and Tribes. The United States assumed this responsibility through a series of treaties with Tribes, exchanging compensation and benefits for Tribal land and peace. The Snyder Act of 1921 (25 USC 13) legislatively affirmed this trust responsibility. To facilitate upholding its responsibility, the federal government created the Indian Health Service (IHS) and tasked the agency with providing health services to AI/ANs. Since its creation in 1955, IHS has worked to fulfill the federal promise to provide health care to Native people.

To provide context for this discussion, I would first like to provide you with some health statistics for American Indians and Alaska Natives (AI/ANs). The AI/AN life expectancy is 4.5 years less than the rate for the U.S. all races population. AI/ANs suffer disproportionally from a variety of diseases. According to IHS data from 2005–2007, AI/AN people die at higher rates than other Americans from alcoholism (552 percent higher), unintentional injuries (138 percent higher), homicide (83 percent higher) and suicide (74 percent higher). Indian Country also suffers disproportionately from diabetes at a rate 182 percent higher than the general U.S. population.

Chronic poverty, historical trauma, remote locations, and a devastatingly underfunded Indian health delivery system all contribute to these statistics. The United States is too great a nation to stand idly by while AI/ANs, the first Americans, live with these realities.

Diabetes in Indian Country

American Indian and Alaska Native (AI/AN) youth, children, and families face many disparate adverse experiences and health outcomes compared to the general U.S. population. One of the most prominent health disparities in Tribal communities is the high rate of type 2 diabetes. AI/ANs of all ages are disproportionately impacted by type 2 diabetes and its many chronic complications- whether through their own individual diagnosis or the diagnosis of a loved one. The Gila River Indian Community has reported a 4 year old presenting with type 2 diabetes—and they are not alone. As such, Tribal communities must have the resources and support they need to access fresh and nutritious foods, safe places for physical activity, and quality diabetes treatment and intervention programs.

Because AI/AN traditional subsistence lifestyles have been replaced with federal programs such as the Food Distribution Program on Indian Reservations, the Food Stamp Program, and the Commodity Supplemental Food Program, many Tribal communities have a new reliance on store-bought foods, poor access to fresh produce, and have increased consumption of fast foods. These compounding issues have resulted in American Indian and Alaska Native children suffering from higher rates of obesity and related complications, such as type 2 diabetes. [1]

Even in the general U.S. population, type 2 diabetes is increasingly diagnosed in youth and now accounts for 20–50 percent of new-onset diabetes case patients. However, type 2 diabetes disproportionately affects minority race and ethnic groups— with the highest rates being among American Indian and Alaska Native youth. While few longitudinal studies have been conducted, it has been suggested that the increase in type 2 diabetes in youth is a result of an increase in obesity in the overall population. [2] The majority of studies that have been done have been conducted on American and Canadian Indigenous populations because of the high rates of diabetes experienced in Tribal communities. Therefore, we know American Indian and Alaska Native youth age 10–19 are nine times more likely to have diagnosed type 2 diabetes compared to young non-Hispanic whites in the same age group. [3] Further-

---

[1] Story, M. et al. (2003). Obesity in American-Indian Children: Prevalence, Consequences, and Prevention. *Preventative Medicine*, 37(1), S3–S12, S5.

[2] (Dabelea, et al., 2014) (2)

[3] SEARCH for Diabetes in Youth Study *http://www.ncbi.nlm.nih.gov/pubmed/17015542*

more, from 1990–2009 AI/AN youth age 15–19 experienced an increase in diagnosed diabetes of 110 percent.[4] While these statistics are staggering, there are personal stories and real life implications behind each of the Native youth and families that have been diagnosed with type 2 diabetes. People with diabetes diagnosed before the age of 20 years have a life expectancy that is 15–27 years shorter than people without diabetes.[5] Given this, it is more important than ever that Tribal communities work to prevent diabetes and its complications in young American Indians and Alaska Natives. One program in particular, the Special Diabetes Program for Indians (SDPI), has been especially successful in establishing and sustaining effective diabetes treatment and prevention programs in Indian Country.

Special Diabetes Program for Indians

Because of the rising rates of type 2 diabetes in American Indian and Alaska Native youth and the U.S. population in general, Congress established the Special Diabetes Program for Indians in 1997. The SDPI was first funded through the Balanced Budget Act in conjunction with the Special Diabetes Program for Type 1 Diabetes (SDP)—a program that addresses the opportunities in type 1 diabetes research. Together, these two programs have become the nation's most strategic, comprehensive and effective effort to combat diabetes and its complications.

The SDPI is changing the troubling statistics for American Indians and Alaska Natives of all ages with marked and measurable improvements in average blood sugar levels, reductions in the incidence of cardiovascular disease, prevention and weight management programs for our youth, and a significant increase in the promotion of healthy lifestyle behaviors. This success is due to the nature of this grant program that allows communities to design and implement diabetes interventions that address specific cultural approaches identified community priorities. The SDPI currently provides grants for over 300 programs in 35 states.

As a result of intensive data collection and analysis over the past two decades of the SDPI, we are able to demonstrate remarkable outcomes from SDPI programs, including a reduction in A1C levels, reduced cholesterol levels, and weight loss of program participants around Indian Country. Recently, the Centers for Disease Control and Prevention (CDC) published data in its Morbidity and Mortality Weekly Report about the remarkable decline in End-Stage Renal Disease (ESRD) due to diabetes seen in American Indians and Alaska Natives in 1996–2013. During this time period, similar to that of the SDPI, AI/ANs have experienced a 54 percent decline in incidence rates of ESRD due to diabetes—the steepest decline of any other ethnic group. The CDC report also states, "because of SDPI, the partnership of IHS and I/T/U programs is stronger, and together they provide a comprehensive public health-oriented national program that has demonstrated success in addressing the diabetes epidemic and reducing complications such as ESRD–D."[6] ESRD treatment costs Medicare roughly $87,000 per patient, per year, so SDPI is also resulting in significant cost savings for federal health programs.[7]

As the data shows, the diabetes treatment and prevention programs funded by SDPI are clearly improving, as well as saving lives, in Tribal communities and transforming the way diabetes is addressed. For example, the Alaska Native Tribal Health Consortium's (ANTHC) "Store Outside Your Door" program highlights traditional foods of the Native peoples living within the region and teaches families how to harvest and prepare nutritious traditional foods that do not include many of the preservatives and sugars of the processed foods often available at local grocery stores. This model makes nutritious foods accessible to the community and infuses the local Indigenous culture back into mealtime. Another example of the effective, innovative community health programming being conducted in Tribal communities around Indian Country is the "Cherokee Choices" program at the Eastern Band of Cherokee Indians (EBCI). Like many Tribal communities, the EBCI has higher rates of obesity and type 2 diabetes than the U.S. general population. To combat these high rates, the Cherokee Choices program includes three main components: elementary school mentoring, worksite wellness for adults, and church-based health promotion.[8] As a holistic approach to preventing diabetes and obesity in the local AI/AN population, Cherokee Choices also seeks to address racism, historic grief and

---

[4] IHS Division of Diabetes Statistics *https://www.ihs.gov/sdpi/includes/themes/newihstheme/display_objects/documents/factsheets/Fact_sheet_AIAN_508c.pdf*

[5] (Mayer-Davis, et al., 2009)

[6] (Bullock, et al., 2017)

[7] U.S. Renal Data System: *https://www.usrds.org/2013/view/v2_11.aspx*, Accessed on March 27, 2017.

[8] Bachar JJ, Lefler LJ, Reed L, McCoy T, Bailey R, Bell R. Cherokee Choices: a diabetes prevention program for American Indians. Prev Chronic Dis [serial online] 2006 Jul [date cited]. Available from: URL: *http://www.cdc.gov/pcd/issues/2006/jul/05_0221.htm*

trauma, mental health, and creates a supportive environment for developing positive policy changes.

These are just two examples of the over 300 Tribal programs nationwide taking an innovative, holistic and community- and evidenced-based approach to preventing diabetes in Native youth, children and families. As one young American Indian from the Klamath Diabetes Program stated after participating in the diabetes prevention program at the Cow Creek Consortium in Oregon, "I truly believe [SDPI] can dramatically improve the health of the Klamath Tribes and bring us mo ben dic hosintambiek ("good health" in Klamath). I would have never had the courage or been in the shape necessary to accomplish my goals had it not been for the Diabetes Prevention Program. It is imperative that these types of programs are firmly in place to lead us to the next level of good health".

Most recently in the long history of the SDPI, in April 14, 2015, the U.S. Senate passed a two year reauthorization of the Special Diabetes Program for Indians (SDPI) as part of The Medicare Access and Children's Health Insurance Program (CHIP) Reauthorization Act of 2015 (P.L. 114–10). The measure passed the Senate by a bipartisan vote of 92–8. This followed action by the U.S. House of Representatives on March 26, 2015, which also passed the legislation by a bipartisan vote. SDPI is one of many programs in this legislation. However, the reauthorization is set to expire on September 30, 2017. Meaning, over 300 diabetes treatment and prevention programs around the country would no longer be available to the most vulnerable population for this devastating disease. Congress must act swiftly to reauthorize the SDPI and ensure continuity in the successful prevention and intervention efforts being conducted all across Indian Country.

NIHB and Tribes are encouraged by the strong support enjoyed by SDPI in Congress. In September 2016, a letter addressed to Congressional leadership in support of SDPI and SDP garnered signatures from 356 House Members and 75 Senators. We hope that Congressional leaders make the renewal of these programs a legislative priority in the coming months. Failure to enact SDPI swiftly will result in the loss of staff for many SDPI programs living in rural areas and will cause disruptions to patient care.

Putting First Kids 1st

The National Indian Health Board, in partnership with the National Congress of American Indians, the National Indian Education Association, and the National Indian Child Welfare Association have created a joint policy agenda for American Indian and Alaska Native children. This agenda, updated in 2015, is intended to be a tool to develop integrated policy approaches and specific recommendations for Tribal governments, policymakers, and local leaders to use when creating and implementing a vision for thriving, vibrant Native communities. The agenda includes a "Healthy Lifestyles" component that outlines policy recommendations that would specifically help policymakers and Tribal communities prevent diabetes in Native youth, children, and families through increasing physical activity, improving access to nutritious foods, and increasing access to health care and public health services. [9] In addition to the swift reauthorization of the Special Diabetes Program for Indians outlined earlier, the NIHB puts forth the following recommendations for Tribes and policymakers to pursue to strengthen diabetes prevention efforts and to make healthy lifestyles more accessible to Native youth and families:

- Ensure that community food programs, especially youth breakfast and lunch programs, incorporate healthy food choices and locally produced or traditional food options.
- Co-locate food assistance programs to serve meals to elders along with Head Start, child care, or school programs to reduce administrative costs and resources.
- Work to improve the Food Distribution Program on Indian Reservations by incorporating more traditional, locally-produced foods as healthier options.
- Provide direct funding to Tribes who want to administer the Supplemental Nutrition Assistance Program (formerly the Food Stamp Program).
- Work to create similar options for the Women, Infants and Children (WIC) program and increase Tribal flexibility in administering this program.
- Advocate for Tribal provisions within the National School Lunch Program and the School Breakfast Program for Tribal schools.

---

[9] Native Children's Policy Agenda: Putting First Kids 1st *http://nihb.org/docs/10122015/ Aug_2015_Native_Childrens_Policy_Agenda.pdf*

- Work with school nutrition programs to replace junk foods with healthier options in vending machines and school cafeterias. These programs should permit Tribal administration and should ensure that state-administered programs are sufficiently responsive to the needs of Native youth.
- Promote the expansion of retail grocery markets in Native communities.
- Support federal programs that encourage at-home food production, such as backyard gardens and training on planting and maintenance.
- Work to ensure that Bureau of Indian Education (BIE) schools receive funding to build and upgrade sports-related facilities, such as gymnasiums, fields, and tracks to increase safe places for Native children and youth to be physically active.
- Incorporate wellness programs in health clinics and facilities. While health care addresses disease prevention and treatment, wellness encompasses daily lifestyle choices, environment, emotional and spiritual well-being, and health education. Through wellness promotion, the incidence of health problems can be reduced, along with long term health care costs.
- Improve outreach services and health education. For example, a Tribal diabetes patient education program, which focuses on teaching people how to manage their disease on a daily basis, is an important tool for reducing diabetes-related complications. These programs can also be directed to helping children manage their diabetes from an early age. Similarly, community outreach services can help educate people about the availability of health benefits and teach children to make healthy choices early in life.
- Develop school-based health clinics. Students perform better in class when they are healthy and ready to learn. School-based health centers bring the doctor's office to the school so students avoid health-related absences and get support to succeed in the classroom.

Conclusion

Thank you again for the opportunity to offer this written statement. While Tribes have made important gains in recent years in terms of type 2 diabetes funding, improved health outcomes, and the leveling off of diabetes incidence rates, there is still a long way to go before Native youth, children, and families will no longer be devastated by the impacts of diabetes and its complications.

The CHAIRMAN. Thank you, Mr. Hawley.
Mr. Eagle.

STATEMENT OF JARED EAGLE, DIRECTOR, FORT BERTHOLD DIABETES PROGRAM, THREE AFFILIATED TRIBES

Mr. EAGLE. Good afternoon, Committee, and Chairman Hoeven. Thank you for the opportunity to speak.

My name is Jared Eagle. I am a member of the Three Affiliated Tribes, the Mandan, Hidatsa, and Arikara Nation.

We serve the people of the Three Affiliated Tribes. We have benefitted SDPI funding for the last 18 years, 15 of those mainly in the clinical format with the last three being in the preventative aspects of it, specifically on youth.

I cannot express enough the importance of the SDPI initiative and the resources that it provides to our community. Through SDPI funding, we have been able to provide essential treatment and prevention initiatives to our over 750 diagnosed patients and provide prevention services to over 1,200 youth based through five schools and about 250 square miles.

The focus of our program is to provide access to effective nutrition and physical activity opportunities that are not accessible to the people on our reservation in most aspects. These initiatives include group fitness classes, cooking classes, grocery store tours, one-on-one dietitian consultation, and prevention resources through screening and education.

We live in a food desert. Of the six communities, we only have two grocery stores in those two communities so access to fresh produce and healthy foods is very minimal sometimes. The overweight and obesity rates on Fort Berthold are 55 percent among youth grades K–12. The adult population is about 86 percent overweight and obese.

The direct link between overweight, obesity and diabetes prevalence, specifically in Native Americans, and the importance of SDPI programming could not be more evident for us.

One major aspect that we incorporate to combat this epidemic which affects about 15 percent the MHA Nation is our Healthy Futures Program. Through Healthy Futures, we screen 1,200 youth in grades K–12 to identify if they are in an overweight or obese status. We identify what their Body Mass Index is. We screen them; for diabetes, and if they show signs of being pre-diabetic, they are referred to a more intense follow-up service with a pediatrician and our clinical staff.

Through this process ,we are able to connect directly with the parents to make the necessary changes to develop and instill healthy behaviors and to avoid a lifestyle of chronic disease.

The work we do at the Fort Berthold Diabetes Program allows us to connect with the communities, and provides us the opportunity to reach a broad demographic of people that our IHS clinic or another hospital simply cannot reach outside of a traditional medical practice.

Culturally, we are able to create deep and lasting connections as well as providing services such as traditional food education, gardening, language and educating at powwows. Other community gatherings reach into and across the communities and make a much stronger individual connection to help save lives. Through SDPI funding we are able to provide these types of services to reduce the incidence of diabetes, preserve the health of our people and reduce the long-term health care costs that they could face.

Thank you for allowing me to witness in front of you today. I will answer any questions or provide any additional information you might need.

[The prepared statement of Mr. Eagle follows:]

PREPARED STATEMENT OF JARED EAGLE, DIRECTOR, FORT BERTHOLD DIABETES PROGRAM, THREE AFFILIATED TRIBES

Good afternoon Committee, my name is Jared Eagle, I am the Director of the Fort Berthold Diabetes Program in New Town, ND. We serve the people of the Three Affiliated Tribes, the Mandan, Hidatsa, and Arikara Nation. Our program has benefitted from 18 years of SDPI funding providing essential diabetes related services to our people ranging from clinical care and prevention for the first 15 years and specifically targeted towards prevention initiatives the past three years.

I cannot express enough the importance of the SDPI initiative and the resources that it provides to our community. Through SDPI funding we are able to provide essential treatment and prevention initiatives to our 750 diagnosed patients and over 1,200 youth spread out among our six communities and five schools in a 250 mile radius.

The focus of our program is to provide access to effective nutrition and physical activity opportunities not accessible to the people on our reservation. These initiatives include group fitness classes, cooking classes, grocery store tours, one-on-one dietitian consultation and prevention resources through screening and education.

We live in a food desert, and of the six communities on Fort Berthold only two have grocery stores and access to fresh produce and healthy food options. The overweight and obesity rates on Fort Berthold are 55 percent among youth grades K–12 and 86 percent among the adult population. The direct link between overweight/obesity and diabetes prevalence, specifically in Native Americans, the importance of SDPI programming could not be more evident.

One major aspect that we incorporate to combat this epidemic which effects about 15 percent of the MHA Nation is our Healthy Futures Program. We screen 1,200 youth in grades K–12 to identify if they are overweight or obese. Those with a high Body Mass Index (BMI), are then screened for diabetes, and if they show signs of being pre-diabetic they are referred for more intense follow-up services with a pediatrician and our clinical team. Through this process we are able to connect directly with the parents to start making the necessary changes to develop and instill healthy behaviors to avoid a lifestyle of chronic disease.

The work we do at the Fort Berthold Diabetes Program allows us to connect with the communities, and provides us the opportunity to reach a broad demographic of people that our IHS clinic or another hospital simply cannot reach outside of a traditional medical practice. Culturally, we are able to create deep and lasting connections as well in providing services such as traditional food education, gardening, language and educating at powwows and other community gatherings that reach into and across the communities and make a much stronger individual connection and save lives.

Through SDPI funding we are able to provide these types of services to reduce the incidence of diabetes, preserving the health of our people and reducing the long-term health care costs that they could face. Thank you for allowing me to testify and I would be happy to answer any questions or provide any additional information.

The CHAIRMAN. Thank you, Mr. Eagle. We appreciate it.

Mr. Sensmeier, I understand you are in the Magnificent Seven, is that correct, and you have a new movie coming out entitled Wind River.

Mr. SENSMEIER. That is right.

The CHAIRMAN. Give us a quick once-over about your character in the last movie and what you are going to do in the next movie.

Mr. SENSMEIER. In the Magnificent Seven, I played one of the Seven starring alongside our national spokesperson and club alumni, Mr. Denzel Washington. In Wind River, I star alongside Jeremy Renner, Elizabeth Olsen and Graham Greene. It takes place on the Wind River, Wyoming Reservation. It is a murder mystery. I am not going to tell you too much about that. I will let you go see it.

STATEMENT OF MARTIN SENSMEIER, ACTOR AND AMBASSADOR, BOYS & GIRLS CLUBS OF AMERICA

Mr. SENSMEIER. Chairman Hoeven, Ranking Member Udall, and distinguished members of the Committee, I want to thank you for the opportunity to testify at today's hearing.

[Greeting in Native Language.]

My original name is [phrase in Native Language]. I am from the Eagle Bear Clan of the Tlingit Tribe of Alaska.

As a Native American actor and Native ambassador of Boys & Girls Clubs of America, it is an honor to be here today to advocate for wellness among Native people of all Nations, focusing largely on our youth.

Growing up, I attended the Boys & Girls Club of Alaska and learned early the benefits of a healthy and active lifestyle. Health is not just about physical and medical, it also impacts how young people cope with emotional and mental health.

I am privileged to be an Ambassador for the Boys & Girls Clubs of America and I am a member of the Native Wellness Institute as well as an Ambassador for the Nike N7 Fund. These platforms have provided an opportunity to reach out to more youth and play a role as a mentor and advocate promoting healthy life styles for our Native youth.

As a former Club kid, I can testify to how Boys & Girls Clubs on Native Lands are working to decrease the high rates of diabetes and obesity in Indian communities though physical activities, nutrition, and education.

For 25 years, Boys & Girls Clubs of America has established an enduring presence on Native lands. Currently, there are nearly 200 Boys & Girls Clubs serving over 86,000 Native youth, from over 100 different American Indian, Alaska Native and Hawaiian communities in 27 States.

As the Nation's largest service provider to Native youth, Boys & Girls Clubs in Indian Country are committed to addressing unique to Native lands through increasing culturally relevant and meaningful opportunities.

Healthy eating and being active has always been a major part of my life. I have been so excited to see the partnership between the Boys & Girls Clubs of America, the National Congress of American Indians and the Indian Health Service on programs such as TRAIL to diabetes prevention that is making healthy living an essential part of the club members' experience.

Even more exciting, however, is the IHS funded program that looks to include traditional food in activities so that youth are connecting with their culture as well as keeping their bodies healthy. I have heard directly that some of the clubs' kids are getting introduced to dried moose meat. It is personally one of my favorites.

The TRAIL Program has reached over 14,000 Native youth in communities across our Country, including my home State of Alaska. I would personally like to thank IHS, NCAI, BGCA and Congress for their continued support of this impactful program that encourages healthy habits and resiliency in Native youth.

It has made a profound difference in Indian Country. I have no doubt it will continue to do so as this Committee lends its direct support. Additionally, through BGCA's Healthy Habits program that serves K–12, youth learn to adopt healthy eating habits. The lessons cover dietary guidelines, understanding food labels, strategies to increase food and vegetable consumption and interactive healthy cooking demonstrations.

Roughly 91 percent of participants reported maintaining or improving their nutrition and healthy habits. Successes were achieved through increasing knowledge about healthy nutritional choices, teaching how to identify healthy options in the grocery store and demonstrating healthy meal preparation. This also includes sharing lessons learned with families and community elders.

Additionally, Triple Play, BGCA's comprehensive health and wellness program, strives to improve the health of Club members ages 6 to 18 by increasing their daily physical activity and teaching them good nutrition. This program utilizes three components: mind, body and soul.

The mind component teaches youth to eat smart through the power of choice, calories, vitamins and minerals, the food pyramid and appropriate portion size. The body component boosts Clubs' traditional physical activities to a higher level by providing sports and fitness activities for all youth. The Soul component helps build positive relationships and cooperation among youth and young people.

In addition, Clubs provide programming that incorporates tribal-focused, non-traditional sports, such as cultural dance, canoeing and archery; while nutrition programs incorporate local, cultural foods and culinary customs to ensure kids are moving and eating a balanced, healthy diet. Generations of children currently benefit from investments in programs at Clubs which help them grow into healthy, responsible adults.

I would like to say that the Boys & Girls Clubs of America has been a very integral part of my success. I am directly affected by diabetes. My dad has diabetes. I am proud to use my platform to be a part of this movement to stop diabetes in Indian Country.

Again, I thank the Committee. We appreciate your interest in this critical issue. I am happy to respond to any questions you may have regarding the movies or the movement.

[The prepared statement of Mr. Sensmeier follows:]

PREPARED STATEMENT OF MARTIN SENSMEIER, ACTOR AND AMBASSADOR, BOYS & GIRLS CLUBS OF AMERICA

Chairman Hoeven, Ranking Member Udall, and distinguished members of the Committee, thank you for the opportunity to testify at today's hearing. My name is Martin Sensmeier of Tlingit, Koyukon-Athabascan, and Irish descent. I was raised in a Tlingit Coastal Community in Southeast Alaska and grew up learning and participating in the traditions of my Tribe. As a Native American actor and Native ambassador of Boys & Girls Clubs of America, it is honor to be here today to advocate for wellness among Native people of all Nations, focusing largely on youth.

Growing up, I attended the Boys & Girls Club of Alaska and learned early the benefits of a healthy and active lifestyle. Health is not just about physical and medical, it also impacts how young people cope with emotional and mental health. Throughout my life and career as an actor it has been important to maintain these habits. I am privileged to be an Ambassador for the Boys & Girls Clubs of America and I am a member of the Native Wellness Institute. These platforms have provided an opportunity to reach out to more youth and play a role as a mentor and advocate promoting healthy life styles for our Native youth.

As a former Club kid, I can testify to how Boys & Girls Clubs on Native Lands are working to decrease the high rates of diabetes and obesity in Indian communities though physical activities, nutrition, and education. For 25 years, Boys & Girls Clubs of America has established an enduring presence on Native lands and has committed to improving the capacity of Boys & Girls Clubs to serve these youth. Currently, there are nearly 200 Boys & Girls Clubs serving over 86,000 Native youth, from over 100 different American Indian, Alaska Native and Hawaiian communities in 27 states.

Boys & Girls Clubs of America continues its pledge to assist communities and expand youth development in Indian Country. Such efforts have been demonstrated by the establishment of the Boys & Girls Clubs of America's Native Services in 2013, and growth in national staff, many who are Native themselves, that work across the country to support our Club professionals. As the Nation's largest service provider to Native youth, Boys & Girls Clubs in Indian Country are committed to addressing the challenges and issues unique to Native lands through an increase in opportunities that are culturally relevant and meaningful.

While many Native youth thrive and succeed in life, as a whole they are one of our country's most vulnerable populations. Persistent issues of unemployment, poverty, physical and sexual abuse and a host of other risk factors existing in Indian Country, have created a climate where suicide, alcoholism and drug abuse amongst tribal youth is perpetuated. There are many statistics that paint an alarming portrait of the well-being of Native youth in America today. Because time is limited, I will offer just two that we are here today to discuss.

1. Native American youth have disproportionally high rates of obesity and diabetes relative to the American populations.

2. The rate of type-2 diabetes among AI/AN youth is nearly 3 times the national average.

Research found that 12–19 year-old AI/AN youth participating in a survey consumed fruits, vegetables and dairy products less than once per day, which is below the recommended dietary allowance.

There are multiple factors that have led to the decline in physical activity and poor nutrition habits across our Native lands. On many Native lands, families are likely to purchase foods that are locally accessible, familiar and convenient to prepare, but may be lacking in nutritional value. Youth many not learn the skills and tools to prepare healthy, balanced meals at home. This contributes to obesity, malnutrition related diseases, and a pattern of poor eating habits.

Because of the relationship between diet and obesity, Clubs are promoting healthy eating behaviors that can help decrease the prevalence of obesity. Boys & Girls Clubs on Native Lands provide the greatest opportunity for impact. Boys & Girls Clubs of America's vision is to turn these Clubs into models of wellness, improving the nutrition and health of youth and families in some of our nation's most impoverished communities.

Through programs like the Boys & Girls Clubs of America's Healthy Habits program that serves K–12, our Clubs empower Native youth with the knowledge and resources to adopt healthy eating habits. Healthy Habits provides outcome-driven nutrition education opportunities for Club members, which is critical to improving their health and wellness.

In 2016, 16 Boys & Girls Clubs in Indian Country from across the country representing various tribal communities provided healthy meals and nutrition education utilizing BGCA's Healthy Habits program in a culturally sensitive and age appropriate way. Lessons covered dietary guidelines, understanding food labels, identifying food groups, strategies to increase fruit and vegetable consumption, and interactive healthy meal and snack cooking demonstrations. Clubs reported that, with consistent participation in the program, youth have begun to share new information and healthy eating strategies with their families.

Native Clubs that implemented the Healthy Habits program reported progress made to promote health and wellness among youth and the greater community. Roughly 91 percent of participants reported maintaining or improving their nutrition and healthy habits, specifically 74 percent improved and 17 percent maintained. Successes were achieved through increasing knowledge about healthy nutritional choices, teaching how to identify healthy options in the grocery store and demonstrating healthy meal preparation. This also includes sharing lessons learned with families and community elders.

Other programs like, Triple Play, BGCA's comprehensive health and wellness program, developed in collaboration with the U.S. Department of Health and Human Services, strives to improve the overall health of Club members ages 6–18 by increasing their daily physical activity, teaching them good nutrition and helping them develop healthy relationships. This program utilizes three components, Mind, Body and Soul. The Mind component encourages young people to eat smart through the Healthy Habits program, which covers the power of choice, calories, vitamins and minerals, the food pyramid and appropriate portion size. The Body component boosts Clubs' traditional physical activities to a higher level by providing sports and fitness activities for all youth. Body programs include six daily fitness challenges; teen Sports Clubs focused on leadership development, service and careers in athletics; and Triple Play Games Tournaments, inter-Club sectional tournaments that involve multiple team sports. The Soul component helps build positive relationships and cooperation among young people.

In addition, Clubs provide programming that incorporates tribal-focused, non-traditional sports, such as cultural dance, canoeing and archery; while nutrition programs incorporate local, cultural foods and culinary customs to ensure kids are moving and eating a balanced, healthy diet.

According to the 2013 United States Census, American Indians/Alaska Natives had a higher rate of poverty than any other racial group, which was 29 percent as compared to the national poverty rate of 15 percent. Due to high poverty rates, access to healthy food options may be limited. As such, meals and snacks provided during Club hours may be the only or last meal a child eats during the day.

Over a lifetime, the medical costs associated with childhood obesity are about $19,000 more per child than those for a child of normal weight. [1]

- Every 100 youth Boys & Girls Clubs help develop habits that enable them to maintain a healthy weight, could save as much as $1.9 million in lifetime medical costs.

- According to the Centers for Disease Control and Prevention, 31 percent of Native Youth are obese, a rate 177 percent higher than that of the general population. Whereas only 30 percent of all U.S. youth get physical exercise every day, Boys & Girls Clubs' outcome data reports 60 percent of Native Club youth exercise 5 or more days per week.

For 25 years, Boys & Girls Clubs in Indian Country have proven to be a game-changer for Native youth, by helping them overcome the many societal issues and personal obstacles they face in their communities and home environments. We would not have been nearly as successful without partners like the Indian Health Services and the National Council of American Indians.

Boys & Girls Clubs will continue to play a critical role in breaking a perpetual cycle of extreme poverty, low academic performance, and significant health problems. We envision Native youth on their path to great futures, succeeding in school, becoming community leaders, assuming roles as contributing members of the workforce, and engaging in regular physical activity and good nutrition.

Boys & Girls Clubs in Indian Country have an unprecedented opportunity to help more Native youth to lead sustainable change, while embracing their culture and traditions. We believe generations of children to come will benefit from investments in programs and services, such as Boys & Girls Clubs, that help them grow into responsible adults—and that America stands to gain from the increased productivity and contributions of these future citizens and Native leaders.

Again, thank you to the Committee, we appreciate your interest in this critical issue. We are happy to respond to any questions.

The CHAIRMAN. Thank you, Mr. Sensmeier.

Mr. SENSMEIER. Thank you.

Mr. Villegas and Ms. Seepie.

STATEMENT OF ALTON VILLEGAS, TRIBAL YOUTH, SALT RIVER PIMA–MARICOPA INDIAN COMMUNITY; ACCOMPANIED BY RACHEL SEEPIE, SENIOR FITNESS SPECIALIST, DIABETES SERVICE PROGRAM—HEALTH SERVICE

Mr. VILLEGAS. Good day, everybody. My name is Alton Villegas.

I am 11 years old and going to be turning 12 in December. I am the oldest brother in my family. I have two really good friends Lorenzo Klein Romero and James Upshaw.

I am a member of the Salt River Pima-Maricopa Indian Community. I am a member of the fifth grade at Salt River Elementary School. I like my school very much and my favorite subject is reading. I also like sports like cross country and wrestling.

When I am home, I like to go jumping on my trampoline with my siblings. Soon, because it is almost summer, I get to go swimming.

Last summer I went to a diabetes prevention camp which is funded by the SDPI grant. My mom and my grandma have diabetes. A lot of people in Salt River have diabetes, sadly. I think a lot of people have diabetes because they do not eat healthy and they do not exercise.

I want to be healthy so I went to camp. I wanted to be able to help my mom and my grandma be healthier. I also wanted to show

[1] Finkelstein, E.A., Graham, W.C.K. and Molhotra, R. (2014). "Lifetime Direct Medical Costs of Childhood Obesity," *Pediatrics*, Vol. 133, No. 5, 854–862, *http://pediatrics.aapublications.org/content/133/5/854.short.*

my brothers and sisters how they could be healthier. When I was there, I lost nearly 16 pounds. I am not done.

Camp also helped me make better choices in what I eat and they taught me that playing outside was fun and not boring. When I came home from camp, my family thought I would like to have a hamburger, fries or a pizza but I did not want that or the salt. At the time, I did not eat the salt, I did not eat all of it.

Like Mr. Hoeven said, that is my idea, order a salad. Chicken Caesar is really good. You should go there.

They were very surprised. I remembered eating junk was not okay, but if I did that, the program taught me eating good and exercising, I would lower my sugar and feel better and I did. I cannot wait to go back to camp again this year. I know I will learn more and will have a lot of fun.

I think more kids would learn from the diabetes camp and they can help other people in Salt River to be healthier so they will not be sick.

I would like to invite you to come to Arizona in the summer. We go to camp where it is not so hot. I want you to see our camp.

Thanks for helping me and helping my mom and my grandma.

[The prepared statement of Mr. Villegas follows:]

PREPARED STATEMENT OF ALTON VILLEGAS, TRIBAL YOUTH, SALT RIVER PIMA-MARICOPA INDIAN COMMUNITY; ACCOMPANIED BY RACHEL SEEPIE, SENIOR FITNESS SPECIALIST, DIABETES SERVICE PROGRAM—HEALTH SERVICE

Background

The Salt River Pima-Maricopa Indian Community appreciates the opportunity to provide oral and written testimony to the Senate Select Committee on Indian Affairs on the Special Diabetes Prevention Initiative, particularly relating to prevention of diabetes among Native Youth through Healthy Living.

The Salt River Pima-Maricopa Indian Community (Community) is a federally recognized tribe created by federal Executive Order on June 14, 1879 and is the homeland of two distinct tribes; the Pima—"Onk Akimel O'odham" (River People), and the Maricopa—"Xalychidom Piipaash" (People who live toward the Water). The Community is comprised of 52,600 acres, with 19,000 held as a natural preserve, which are divided into Community-owned land and individual allotments. SRPMIC consists of two geographical areas; the Salt River and Lehi Communities that are separated by the Salt River, with the Lehi Community located south of the river. The Community lands are adjacent to the Phoenix metropolitan area in central Arizona and located within Maricopa County. SRPMIC shares a common boundary with the cities of Mesa, Tempe, and Scottsdale, town of Fountain Hills and Ft. McDowell Yavapai Nation. Current total enrolled membership is 10,378 of which approximately 6,000 members reside within the Community's boundaries.

Unlike many remotely located Indian reservations, SRPMIC lies within a county determined to be one of the most rapidly growing metropolitan populations, which has brought two major commuter freeways to the Community. However, the Community still lags far behind the United States and nearby adjacent cities in both social and economic development and experiences social and health problems similar to those found on more remotely located reservations.

Medical services are provided by a combination of Indian Health Service (Phoenix Indian Medical Center and the Salt River Health Clinic), regional healthcare corporations (Scottsdale Osborn Hospital and Mayo Clinic), and private practice providers located throughout the metropolitan area.

In addition, the Community supports a Department of Health and Human Services (HHS) which provides clinical staff working in coordination with federal providers at the Salt River Health Clinic. Within HHS, there are Public Health workers, Behavioral Health therapists, Prevention and Intervention services, psychiatrists, WIC and other administrative staff. These programs are supported not only with tribal funds but other grant funding.

The Community has over 10,000 enrolled members and approximately 6000 of our members live in Salt River. 39 percent of our members are under age 18. 53 percent of our members are female and 47 percent are male. The five year rolling average age of death for 2016 and the four preceding years is 48.19 years of age for males and 58.09 years of age for females. The highest number of deaths occur in the age group 20–45. Many of the deaths are related to diabetes and its' complications.

Special Diabetes Prevention Initiative in SRPMIC

The Community Council has identified reducing the prevalence of diabetes in the Community as a needed priority. The Council views the prevalence of diabetes and resulting complications as one of the related causes to the early death rates in the Community. The consequence of these early deaths are devastating for the children, families and the Community.

Health issues in the Community have been identified by the elected Community Council, Diabetes Advisory Team (DAT), and obesity screening by the elementary and high school nurses.

Since many of our tribal members and their families receive health care through the Indian Health Service, we are able to pull the following data from the electronic health record system for the time period January 1, 2016—December 31, 2016.

There are 1062 patients from the Salt River Community who are in the Diabetes Registry. We know from the data that there are more females than males who are diabetic and seeking medical care. We also know that the prevalence is highest in the age grouping 45–64 years of age. The diabetics in our Community are almost all Type 2 diabetics who are obese or severely obese with a majority being diagnosed 10+ years ago. There is a high number of these patients who have been diagnosed with hypertension (829) and also some patients diagnosed with cardiovascular disease (277). Almost half of those diagnosed with Type 2, have chronic kidney disease.

> *Gender:* Female = 652; Male = 410
>
> *Age:* <20 yr = 12; 20–44 = 278; 45–64 = 547; 65>= 225
>
> *Type* Type 1 = 1; Type 2 = 1061
>
> *Duration of Diabetes:* Less than 1 year = 33; Less than 10 years = 401; More than 10 years = 467

For those participating in Diabetes treatment, 26 percent use diet and exercise to help control their diabetes. They may also use the diet and exercise in combination with insulin 43 percent or metformin 31 percent.

The SRPMIC Diabetes Services Program, is community based and operates within the Department of Health and Human Services (DHHS) Division of Health Services. The Salt River Health Clinic is a unique partnership between the Indian Health Service Phoenix Indian Medical Center (PIMC) and the DHHS. The Diabetes Services Program collaborates with the SRPMIC Clinic providers to ensure coordination of services, and to address the Community members' need for prevention and treatment at every stage

SDPI—Youth Focus

Approximately 3 years ago we had a 6 year old child diagnosed with Type 2 diabetes and we identified the youngest person being dialyzed was age 25. This situation led to greater partnering with the schools and families to have a greater impact on diabetes diagnoses and prevention.

Screening in the schools revealed that 52 percent of the students are above the 95th percentile for weight demonstrating a critical need for more intervention with children, youth, and their families focusing on increased fitness to reduce the risk for diabetes. The screening data suggests that children's weight begins to dramatically increase by the age of 9.

The following diabetes related health issues also impact the youth:

- The Community experience challenges and barriers for diabetes prevention, including the Community culture.
- Accessing nutritious food is difficult for Community residents.
- Existing diabetes intervention services need to be expanded.
- Programs do not always reach the people that need the services.
- People need the intervention to fit their needs.

Why the SDPI is Important to the Salt River Pima-Maricopa Indian Community

Innovative Programming

The SDPI grant has afforded several opportunities to the Community to explore innovative approaches to diabetes prevention and intervention that go beyond the traditional nutrition and exercise curricula. The SRPMIC Diabetes Services Program has hosted two instances of Yoga Teacher Training (YTT) in partnership with the non-profit Conscious Community Yoga to create certified yoga instructors. Yoga is a great low-impact introduction to exercise that takes a holistic approach to health and wellness. To date, approximately 12 individuals have completed the YTT and conduct yoga classes within the Department of Corrections (DOC), Journey to Recovery (residential treatment), and at the Fitness Center. Participants at the DOC have seen encouraging outcomes related to blood pressure and an increased general sense of calmness. Interestingly, the DOC program has a higher attendance from the male population than the female population.

More recently, the SRPMIC Diabetes Services Program is sponsoring a traditional Chinese medicine (TCM) approach to health and wellness called the 5 Elements Wellness Program. The Community has partnered with a local TCM practitioner, Dr. Qingsong Xiao, to conduct a 12-week program that includes exercise, wellness education, herbal supplements and acupuncture. Participants report incredible outcomes that include several point decreases in A1c readings, an increase in energy and activity level, better and more consistent sleep, and weight loss. This has become a very popular program within the Community, and HHS has included a children's component to the program that started at the end of February, 2017.

Collaborations with Women, Infants and Children (WIC) and the School

The Diabetes Program partners with other programs to reach all ages of the Community. The WIC supervisor has a team of four that works with families to educate on the importance of breastfeeding, preparing and eating nutritious meals and managing gestational diabetes. The fitness center staff also assist with offering child friendly exercises during FIT WIC sessions so parents learn about the importance of starting physical activity at a young age.

There are two schools on the reservation serving children from pre-school through 12th grade. The Diabetes program has been able to collaborate with the schools in teaching students about eating healthy and staying active. One initiative known as #GetFit, aims to teach student athletes in becoming role models, wellness champions, to fellow students. The program this year was expanded to reach the parents of student athletes and Physical Education students. Through this program families have the opportunity to learn healthy lifestyle behaviors as well as setting healthy goals as a family.

The Diabetes Camp

The American Indian Youth Wellness (Diabetes Prevention) Camp was established in 1991. Through a collaborative partnership with the University of Arizona and other tribes these one week camps are continuing to be offered. Salt River Pima-Maricopa Indian Community has been participating in camp since the mid 1900's. Every summer in June, the Diabetes Program has been able to pay for and send 20 students and 8 volunteers to camp. The camp involves American Indian youth from tribes across the Southwest, primarily Arizona, to a one week intensive residential camp. At camp, kids learn healthy eating habits and ways to make exercise fun, consistent, and habitual. The best part of camp is that activities take place in an American Indian context, deeply rooted in culture. This integration increases our effectiveness and makes health fun.

Community Wellness Activities

Every year the SRPMIC Diabetes Services Program is able to organize and host several walks within the Community to encourage physical fitness and as outreach for the program itself. Families are encouraged to walk together, often you will see not only the parent, but also the grandparent participating. Additionally, the fitness staff are often called upon by other departments to lead warm-up exercises for activities, i.e. the annual Fall Overhaul which is an Administration hosted event as a community service project for employees; collaborate on certain awareness campaigns such as walks for domestic violence, and suicide prevention.

Summary

The Community appreciates the opportunity to provide testimony on the Special Diabetes Prevention Initiative and the impact that it has had on youth wellness. We appreciate the support of Congress in ensuring that the program continues to be available so that our goal of Community wellness can be achieved.

The CHAIRMAN. Thank you, Mr. Villegas, that was very good.
Ms. Seepie.
Ms. SEEPIE. Good afternoon, Chairman Hoeven, Vice Chairman Udall and members of the Committee.

My name is Rachel Seepie and I am a member of the Salt River Pima-Maricopa Indian Community in Arizona.

It is an honor to appear before you to share my personal journey and let you know how important SDPI has been for me and many members of the community. My community, the Salt River Pima-Maricopa Indian Community, has over 10,000 enrolled members; approximately 6,000 members live within the borders of the community.

Demographically in our community, nearly 40 percent of our members are under the age of 18. By gender, 53 percent of our members are female, 47 percent are male. As you may be aware, the Pima have been the subject of national surveys, news pieces and other studies documenting the high rate of diabetes that exists.

For example, the five-year rolling average age of death of our community for 2016 was 48 years old for male and 58 years old for female. Many of these deaths are directly related to diabetes and its complications.

For many years, the SDPI grant has approved a program for the Committee to give nutritional education and physical activity to prevent diabetes and help those with Type 2 diabetes to lead a healthier lifestyle. I believe with continuation of the grant, more community members of the Salt River Pima-Maricopa Indian Community will learn what is needed to have a healthier lifestyle.

In my own experience, the program has helped me strive to have a healthier life. I am the mother of three children. I learned through the years that physical activity is the key to staying healthy with Type 2 diabetes. Yes, I do have Type 2 diabetes. I have been controlling my Type 2 diabetes with eating well and exercising.

When I was first diagnosed with Type 2 diabetes, I did take medication to control my diabetes. At one time, I decided that I did not want to take medication anymore. I used what I learned from our program in our community to control my diabetes, healthy eating and physical activity. Some of the physical activities I am involved in are aerobic exercise classes, hiking, and running long distance triathlons. For the past ten years, I have run six marathons, 10 half marathons and many triathlons.

The personal achievement I am most proud of is finishing two Iron Man triathlons. I will always remember when I crossed the finish line after swimming 2.4 miles, biking 112 miles and running a marathon which is 26.2 miles, the announcer saying, you are an Iron Man. I heard that twice.

I am also involved in teaching group exercise classes for both youth and seniors in my community. As a result, I have felt healthier and hopefully the people who come to my classes feel healthier also.

I see my doctor and I have positive results. My blood sugar levels have gone down to near normal. My heart rate is low, which means my heart is healthy and strong and I have lost weight myself.

I believe because of the SDPI grant I have more information I need to take care of myself and my family and to live a healthier life so my children can live their lives without Type 2 diabetes.

My vision is that the Salt River Pima-Maricopa Indian Community and our members will learn how to become healthier and that they will have long, full lives without Type 2 diabetes.

Thank you for allowing me to share these few words. I am happy to answer any questions.

The CHAIRMAN. Ms. Seepie, your record running marathons and the Iron Man contest is remarkable.

Ms. SEEPIE. Thank you.

The CHAIRMAN. An amazing achievement and very impressive.

Again, we appreciate all of our witnesses very much. At this time, I will turn to Senator Murkowski.

Senator MURKOWSKI. Thank you, Chairman Hoeven. I appreciate it.

Thank you to all of our panelists. I think in so many different ways, you each are such significant role models for others. Some may be doing it in a more high-profile way, like you, Martin, or perhaps Alton, it is what you can do as you go back to your classroom and talk to other kids about why it is important to each healthy.

The lessons that have shared with us today are all very real takeaways that can make a difference. I think we recognize that so much of this is education. We have talked about the significance of the SDPI program and all that is.

Education only goes so far. You have to act on it and take that step to do the exercise. You have to take that step to order the salad. You have to be proactive with it.

Martin, I noted that it was not too long ago that you flew back up to Juneau to attend the Gold Medal Basketball Tournament that is going on there. Again, it is one of these things where you are flying incredible distances to go to be somewhere where I guess you probably did really love basketball growing up in Yakutat but the fact of the matter is this gives you an opportunity to role model for these other kids so that they see that exercise can be fun.

Can you speak a little bit to this whole aspect of being the role model to get others to be motivated and change behavior because I think this is such an important part of what we are trying to do here.

Mr. SENSMEIER. Yes, we got a gold medal. I think it is one of the oldest, if not the oldest, tournament in the United States, the 71st annual tournament this year. I grew up going. My dad took me. My dad was a Golden Gloves boxer and he started taking me to Gold Medal when I was eight years old.

Basketball has actually become a part of our culture. Physical fitness has always been a big part of my life.

Growing up and attending the Boys & Girls Club, I always had access to that. I had good role models there I looked up to and also mentors who encouraged me to dream big. I was always taught that physical fitness and applying myself, learning nutritional education and all those things that were provided through the clubs would help me get to the level where I am today. I believe that.

There is a quote by Kevin Spacey that says if you should be so lucky to make it to the top, it is your duty to send the elevator back down. I think given the platform I have been blessed to have, I feel it is important, it is a responsibility to promote healthy and active lifestyles in our communities to prevent diabetes and other issues we are dealing with.

Senator MURKOWSKI. We appreciate your leadership and that role modeling that goes on.

I was struck, Mr. Eagle, with your testimony coming from Fort Berthold. You talked about lack of access to healthy foods, the fact that in your reservation stores, available fresh produce is limited.

It strikes me that you are in very much the same situation we have up north in Alaska where 80 percent of our communities are not connected by road, so you have food that is flown in and it is expensive, if you can get it.

Quite honestly, oftentimes it has been sitting somewhere for a long period of time. By the time it gets to the main hub and gets out to the village, if it is lettuce, it is brown, wilted, or dead and nothing that anyone would want to eat.

Kids do not know what color a banana should really look like because by the time it gets to a village, it is really not fit for consumption. So many of our kids have grown up not only not tasting these good, healthy foods, but if they are able to taste it, they are bad by then so they do not like it.

When we think about the education we are building, that is great but we also have to be able to have the access. I know that through USDA and FDA, we have allowed our schools in Alaska, several of our village schools, to accept donated traditional foods that can be served as part of the school lunch menu.

You are having good fish. They are making fish soup instead of opening a can of chili made somewhere else and loaded with preservatives and whatever they load it with. Making sure we have access to the good, healthy traditional foods I think is so important.

We also need to make sure that again we have a way to help get the good food available at an affordable price. We do have our programs out there through SNAP and some of the others, but I look at the connection between the debilitating disease that can be arrested if we are able to focus on diet and exercise.

If we cannot make that good food available, we are still very, very challenged. Know this is something I want to continue to work on with the Committee. We have things like essential air service that help us lower our prices for food. That is on the budget floor right now. It is something we have to address. That is a subject for another time.

Thank you, Mr. Chairman.

The CHAIRMAN. Senator Murkowski, you are right. I agree.

Senator Franken.

Senator FRANKEN. Thank you, Mr. Chairman, again.

As I said in my opening, I have been working on the fight against diabetes since I got here. I, along with Senator Lugar of Indiana, got the National Diabetes Prevention Program into the ACA. It is a program that works with people who are pre-diabetic and their glucose levels are elevated. It gives them 16 weeks of training in both exercise and physical training and 16 weeks in nutritional training. It works.

It has been demonstrated to work. It especially works in older people who are pre-diabetic. They are 70 percent less likely to become diabetic in the next five years if they take the 16-week program. That is why CMS covers it under Medicare if you are on Medicare.

Can you tell me, Admiral, about the programs in IHS and how the Indian direct program may differ? Are you familiar with the National Diabetes Prevention Program?

Mr. BUCHANAN. I am not familiar.

Senator FRANKEN. It is something that WISE did with the CDC. It is 16 weeks of nutritional training accompanied with 16 weeks of physical training. What is the program in Indian Country?

Mr. BUCHANAN. The program in Indian Country takes a holistic approach as was mentioned earlier in some of our discussions. Some of the ideas that were mentioned related to education, physical activity, those sorts of things. We cannot forget social economics that play a big part in this.

Senator FRANKEN. Is there a protocol? Is there a specific protocol?

Mr. BUCHANAN. Could you ask the question again?

Senator FRANKEN. Is there a specific protocol to the program? In other words, the National Diabetes Prevention Program has 16 weeks of physical training and then nutritional training. I know it encompasses those elements of nutrition and exercise.

I was wondering is there a period of time in which it is taught?

Mr. BUCHANAN. With the special diabetes program, we accept applications and it is based on the submissions from the applicants. We have tool kits that are developed and utilized. We utilize best practices we learned as described in some of the testimony provided earlier. It is really a community-based program.

Senator FRANKEN. It is different for each area?

Mr. BUCHANAN. Correct.

Senator FRANKEN. I understand.

A few years ago, I was not in Salt River, but I was in Gila River and they have a resort there that at the time had the best golf course in the Starwood system and the only five-star restaurant in Arizona.

They showed me around their hospital, which was a great state-of-the-art hospital. But they pointed me to three out buildings, I think it was three, and they said those are our dialysis buildings.

They have a five-star restaurant at the resort which is like 15 miles from where everyone lives, but where everyone lives is a food desert. I just think that is an enormous issue. It is hard to eat well when that food is not available. Every time I see them, the Gila River folks, I ask them what is going on with that.

It just seems if you have a five-star restaurant 15 miles away, wherever you are getting that produce at the five-star restaurant, you can get some of it to where you live. I was wondering if anyone had any comments on that. Mr. Eagle?

Mr. EAGLE. Maybe I am answering your question wrong as well but as far as SDPI goes and best practices. Those best practices allow us to do a multidimensional array of things from grocery store tours to having DPP. We run DPP in our program.

Senator FRANKEN. You do?

Mr. EAGLE. It is through collaboration with the North Dakota Health Department, with our local IHS and we utilize the TRAIL Program with the Boys & Girls Clubs. We use that program in our schools and have been doing that for over ten years and we are not a Boys & Girls Club.

SDPI allows us to be very multidimensional and to reach all those different aspects that meet the needs of our people. As you said, nothing is the same in Utah or Montana. Nothing is the same in Fort Berthold as it is in Spirit Lake or Belcort. We are all a bit different. You meet the needs of your people through the services they want to see.

Senator FRANKEN. Right. Thank you, Mr. Eagle.

Thank you.

The CHAIRMAN. Senator Heitkamp.

STATEMENT OF HON. HEIDI HEITKAMP,
U.S. SENATOR FROM NORTH DAKOTA

Senator HEITKAMP. Thank you, Mr. Chairman and Vice Chairman Udall for having this hearing.

One thing I want to examine is the intersection of diabetes prevention with behavior and mental health and the complications that having other challenges in communities presents beyond food deserts.

When someone is suffering from chronic depression, it is not likely they are going to be compliant or even capable maybe at that point in their life of doing the great work that our witnesses talked about today, running a triathlon or educating a whole family about the value of nutrition.

I would like to talk a bit about how we can do a better job holistically because I think when we just focus on one piece, we miss the rest. For instance, some of the highest rates of tobacco usage in my State are in Indian Country. You know this, Jared.

How do we incorporate broadly additional programs to meet all the challenges that I think would maybe achieve better results? We will start with you, Admiral.

Mr. BUCHANAN. In 1997, when the program first started, IHS awarded $30 million. Thirty percent of our facilities had diabetes clinical program teams. Since that time, in 2004, we were currently funded at $115 million, that number went up well above 97 percent.

The diabetes clinical program team can vary depending on the resources available and those sorts of things with physicians, nurses and behavioral health specialists being a part of that team and taking that holistic approach.

We have come a long way from 1997 to now. Continuing that with some of the best practices is an approach forward.

Senator HEITKAMP. Vinton?

Mr. HAWLEY. Building public health systems within tribes would definitely help assist tribes with behavioral health issues. I think with SDPI, it also gives the tribes, as Mr. Eagle stated, the ability to create that infrastructure for your own tribe cultural competency.

If you are encompassing your needs of your tribe and the needs of your people based on your cultural relevancy because we are all different, we are not all the same, we are not all in the same areas and we do our own issues within our own regions, I think with

SDPI, it gives tribes the ability to look at your culture and incorporate it.

When you are incorporating those areas within diabetes, all of those cultural components are also covered in behavioral health issues. It gives you a sense of identity, a sense of well being, a sense of this is who I am, this is where I am from. This is historically what our people did that allowed us to live within ourselves, within our communities and also to live healthy.

I think it encompasses a lot when you talk about behavioral health and the ability to be well, live well, and live healthy and incorporate it. That is a unique thing with SDPI and behavioral health because that is another component that all tribes across the Nation have serious issues with. That encompasses a lot. Thank you for the question.

Senator HEITKAMP. Jared?

Mr. EAGLE. I know I can specifically speak for the work that we do in Fort Berthold but as Senator Murkowski and you just said, we need to work on getting those food deserts access.

I think there is another piece though with behavioral health in the work that we do with SDPI. That is teaching people how to manage when you do not have it. From the example in my testimony, two of the six communities on Fort Berthold have grocery stores. The other four do not. They have access to a convenience store where you can buy chips and pop.

One of our local convenience stores is actually the leader in the State of North Dakota per capita for chip sales. It is a community of less than 700. That says something.

Through SDPI, we try to focus on that behavior because it is a decision to buy what you are buying. If it is not there, yes, that is a major obstacle I agree but there are ways to change that behavior into what is a better option.

All those things are looked at through the different curricula that we utilize such as TRAIL and DPP. In all the activities we do, it is addressed in some form, but not specifically with a mental health provider.

Senator HEITKAMP. I think my point was that siloing just has not worked.

Mr. EAGLE. Yes.

Senator HEITKAMP. It is like saying we are going to fix problems with youth challenges simply with the housing program and ignoring education and health care. This needs to be a collaborative effort.

It is good to hear that this program actually encourages the integration and expansion into behavioral health but we need to do a better job.

The CHAIRMAN. Thank you, Senator Heitkamp.

Admiral, my question for you is we are seeing a decrease in adults but not in youth in terms of both the diabetes and obesity rates. Why is that and what do we need to do?

Mr. BUCHANAN. We are seeing an increase in youth?

The CHAIRMAN. My understanding is we are seeing a decline in the rates for adults but not so with youth. Why is that and what can we do?

Mr. BUCHANAN. The youth rate is leveling off for sure. The Special Diabetes Program has had a tremendous impact over the last 20 years. We are utilizing those lessons learned and best practices going forward to address the youth. Of 301 grantees, 252 are tribal programs. We are utilizing some of those best practices to address the youth.

The CHAIRMAN. Are there changes, improvements or recommendations that you would make to the program? Are there performance measures that should be employed?

Mr. BUCHANAN. With the Special Diabetes Program enacted by Congress, we are reporting on an annual basis on the outcomes related to the diabetes program. We are happy to work with the Committee going forward.

The CHAIRMAN. Are there recommendations you would make for changes or improvements to the program?

Mr. BUCHANAN. Changes or improvements, we a have a Tribal Leaders Diabetes Committee that is an advisory committee to the director. Any significant changes that happen through the program, we work through the Tribal Leaders Diabetes Committee to provide recommendations to the director. The activities up to this point have been recommendations from that committee.

The CHAIRMAN. Mr. Hawley, how could the SDPI program be improved to help further reduce youth obesity and diabetes rates in tribal communities?

Mr. HAWLEY. I think overall is the education and public health. I think the public health is an important tool that can be utilized to educate. In the testimony, I talked a bit about how much more tribal youth are aware than I was when I was in high school of anything that goes on, and the things they are exposed nowadays is beyond anything I remember. I just cannot believe they are aware of some of the things they are aware of and their ability to be engaged, to overcome and get involved, and get active.

That also is our responsibility to show them and encourage, educate and promote. I think that is the key. We have some activities outside of the regular work but then you also have the individuals who are managing these programs even at the national level who are advocating.

However, you also have the individuals who are doing things outside on their own time throughout the week to be engaged, educate and convey the message that we are advocating at this level.

I think it goes a long way when you talk about what we can do to change. As a tribal leader, I know reductions say a lot and raises flags for tribal leaders because we think about tribes doing more with less. We have always done that, I think.

When we talk about those things, the first thing that comes to my mind is how are we going to do more with less because we have done it before and that is what we are going to have to do again but also educating our youth to be active, engaged and the voice of change.

We heard the testimony from the young man down the table and what they are able to accomplish. This is one 11-year old. When that changes throughout Indian Country, it says a lot for the activities. I think it starts with education.

The CHAIRMAN. Mr. Eagle, I am very impressed with the variety of things you are doing. It speaks to the flexibility of the program which is encouraging. Are there other things that you think would be helpful as we work to reauthorize this program, things we should be looking to try to do?

Mr. EAGLE. One thing I guess comes to my mind immediately when it comes to change would be what Vice Chairman Udall said in his opening remarks about continuation funding. The previous example from the kidney report they did and the correlation between SDPI starting and how those rates have declined in conjunction with SDPI funding. That has been done, like you said in a one to two-year reapplication process.

The CHAIRMAN. Right.

Mr. EAGLE. What would happen if this was funded for several years, we had this funding and were able to make plans and do that kind of work on a long-term basis?

The CHAIRMAN. The idea of reauthorizing for a longer period of time and then even maybe carry over funds or something like that would help you, create continuity in your programs and strengthen them?

Mr. EAGLE. Absolutely.

The CHAIRMAN. I will pause here and turn to the Vice Chairman.

Senator UDALL. Thank you, Mr. Chairman.

SDPI is an excellent example of the difference investing in preventative care can make for whole communities. All of you, in a way, have demonstrated that. Unfortunately, this Committee hears from Native constituents that access to preventative and specialty care remains limited in Indian Country.

Admiral, this is for you. In fiscal year 2017, how many Indian Health Service areas can fund, purchase and refer care above medical priority Level 1?

Mr. BUCHANAN. That is a great question. All of our facilities should at least fund between Level 1 in all PRC programs.

Senator UDALL. All of the facilities are doing that now?

Mr. BUCHANAN. That is correct.

Senator UDALL. Where does the money for these preventative services come from, direct appropriations or third party billing from Medicaid and insurance?

Mr. BUCHANAN. I need to back up a little bit.

Senator UDALL. Go ahead.

Mr. BUCHANAN. You were asking for preventative services related to PRC?

Senator UDALL. Yes.

Mr. BUCHANAN. PRC is specifically for the different categories and it goes into different sections from Level 1, Level 2, down to Levels 3 and 4. The preventative piece is farther down. When I was responding, Level 1 is for life and limb types of activity.

Senator UDALL. Right.

Mr. BUCHANAN. I do not have the answer for the preventative piece of it. I can definitely get back to you on that.

Senator UDALL. The point of the question I think was how widespread is the preventative service in all the facilities with SDPI? I think that is what we were trying to get at. You can answer for the record but is it widespread? Is it not in that many areas?

Mr. BUCHANAN. Currently, we have 252 tribal programs. We have about 29 urban programs that are funded and about 15–20 Federal programs funded through SDPI. All those programs, SDPI is all about prevention. Correlating that, we have 782,000 people impacted by the SDPI Program. I hope that answers your question.

Senator UDALL. Is it in every Indian Health Service area?

Mr. BUCHANAN. Thirty-five States. I am hearing my staff say yes, we have SDPI in all of our facilities across the area.

Senator UDALL. The point was made here and several of the witnesses have asked and been asked, we know it is a key to have healthy food but can they access healthy food. To any of you this is kind of a yes or no question.

Those of you living in Indian Country, can you access healthy food in Indian Country or are you living in food deserts? Give me just a yes or no on that. Can you access healthy food? Jared?

Mr. EAGLE. At Forth Berthold, we can. Like said, in limited areas, there are two grocery stores based on a 250-mile radius.

Senator UDALL. It is a lot like the Navajo Reservation where we have 175,000 people over 27,000 square miles and we have ten grocery stores. Is that true in the rest of your communities?

Mr. SENSMEIER. In Alaska, in a lot of the communities there, we have limited access to fresh produce.

Senator UDALL. In your community, Martin, limited access?

Mr. SENSMEIER. It is getting better. You see it is improving but up north, well, my mom comes from the Yukon, it is very limited.

Senator UDALL. Very limited.

Mr. Hawley.

Mr. HAWLEY. Very rural, limited access.

Senator UDALL. Mr. Villegas, do you get that good salad you were talking about earlier there?

Mr. VILLEGAS. Yes.

Senator UDALL. Okay, good. You two are from the same community. Would you agree with that?

Ms. SEEPIE. Yes, we live in an area where we are surrounded by the city, major cities like Scottsdale, Mesa and Phoenix, so we do have access to fresh vegetables and produce.

Senator UDALL. How about on the reservation?

Ms. SEEPIE. On the reservation, we do also have a food bank that does give out fresh fruits and vegetables that community members can also access.

Senator UDALL. Please.

Mr. SENSMEIER. I think on some of the reservations you see failing health but they do have access to fresh produce and stuff like that. It is really helpful when you have programs like Triple Play through the Boys & Girls Clubs of America that educate these young kids about nutrition because one of the biggest problems we have in Indian Country is the lack of nutritional education.

Fried bread, for example, a lot of Native people think fried bread is a Native traditional food. It is not. That was a ration that was given. Now there is a vicious cycle that greatly contributes to diabetes.

When you educate these kids, and break that cycle, then they have a better understanding of how to eat better. Triple Play is one of the great programs. It improves the health of club members ages

6 through 18. The mind component is the biggest one, teaching them to eat smart through the power of choice, calories, vitamins and minerals and appropriate portion size.

I think when we have programs like this our chance of breaking these cycles is a lot greater. My Club rep actually has some really great announcements about that if she can have a chance to speak at some point.

Senator UDALL. Mr. Chairman, I have run over. Thank you.

The CHAIRMAN. Martin, my question kind of goes to a role model in general, not only in terms of healthy eating but in general, good habits, a good lifestyle, how you succeed as a young person and so forth.

For a minute, tell us how you got into acting. It sounds like you had sports and so forth in your background and the Boys & Girls Club but how do you get from that and get into acting particularly at such a high level?

Then talk about it in terms of how you can be a role model or how you get other young people to achieve their dreams? It might be acting or sports or something else for them. Just talk about your own experience for a minute. We are interested to hear, at least I am, how you transitioned to acting and what it took to be successful and what you would advise other young people like maybe Mr. Villegas, to do to achieve their dreams.

Mr. SENSMEIER. It has always been a dream of mine ever since I was a kid. Billy Mills, who was the only American to ever win the 10,000-meter race in the Olympics won in 1964. He was from Pine Ridge Indian Reservation.

I heard him speak one time. He said our children and kids live in a poverty of dreams. They are not allowed to dream; they do not know how to dream. When you encourage them to dream and make them believe in themselves, great things can happen.

I always had that support system through the Club, my parent and role models I saw growing up. That dream was always there. Getting access to be able to make that happen was kind of an unrealistic idea.

I did what a lot of young people do in Alaska. I got into fishing, construction and ended up working on an oil rig. While I was working on the oil rig, I had a lot of time off, two weeks on and two weeks off, so I started traveling to California.

I was like, I am going to check out an acting class. I started getting around other people that were dreaming big. I started seeing people succeed. I was like, okay, I can do this. I stuck with it and stayed persistent and believed in my own ability and started becoming successful.

One of the ways I would like to encourage youth, I try to do my best, is I maintain my connection with the community and make myself accessible to the community. I get a lot of requests to travel around and visit different Native communities all over the Country. I cannot name how many reservations I have been to. I have been in Florida, Connecticut, New York, Washington, Nevada, California, all over the place.

Whether they pay me or not, I try to make myself as accessible as I can. When I am there, I try to promote healthy lifestyles. Senator Murkowski mentioned the Gold Medal tournament in Alaska and I made it a point to go home to that, because everybody at home, all the kids look up to me.

When they see me actively living a healthy lifestyle and also participating in a sporting event, they want to do that too. I wore a Mohawk in the movie and I had ten kids surrounding me and half of them had Mohawks.

I have never set out to be a leader. I do not think of myself as a leader. I think of myself as an example and I strive to be that.

The CHAIRMAN. There is no question you are a leader and that you are having a very powerful, positive impact on your peers and young people. I just want to encourage you to keep it up. Your coming here today shows you care and you are willing to give back. Given where you, that is a remarkable and wonderful thing.

Mr. SENSMEIER. Thank you. I appreciate that.

The CHAIRMAN. Thank you so much.

Mr. Villegas, I am going to turn to you and ask how do you get kids your age tuned in to just what you are doing and talking about? How do you do it? How do you get other people your age to start thinking about health, diet and the right kind of lifestyle as you are doing at a pretty darned young age? Any ideas how you get them interested in it?

Mr. VILLEGAS. I do not know. It is kind of hard.

The CHAIRMAN. It is hard.

Mr. VILLEGAS. Yes.

The CHAIRMAN. Do you talk to them about it?

Mr. VILLEGAS. Yes, I talk to many people about it saying they should really go to the camp and why they should start eating healthy and all that stuff. I tell them all the time but not a lot of people care because they have to give up hot Cheetos.

The CHAIRMAN. Can't they have hot Cheetos once in a while if the rest of the time they are following a really good diet?

Mr. VILLEGAS. No, it is up to them, hot Cheetos, they are addicted to it. I see kids buy at least four bags a day from the ice cream man.

The CHAIRMAN. I think the fact that you are a good example and talking to them about it really does help so I encourage you to keep doing it just as you are today.

Mr. VILLEGAS. There is one thing they have to do to get to that.

The CHAIRMAN. Okay?

Mr. VILLEGAS. We must destroy the ice cream man.

The CHAIRMAN. Okay. We will make sure we get that in the record.

Mr. VILLEGAS. I also think we should have more flyers everywhere saying a good start is to go the camp. Put up a whole bunch of flyers. The reason I found out about the camp was because of a lady named Ms. Mary Lynn. She gave me a flyer and I thought, this sounds like fun and when I was there, I was like, yay, I know how to exercise.

I think that people should know about it and at least consider it and go to the camp. I want to encourage people to go and tell them all the fun stuff that we have.

The CHAIRMAN. That sounds like very good advice. Thank you. Thanks for being here today.

Ms. Seepie, I would ask you the same question that I asked some of the other witnesses. Your record with the training and discipline it takes to run marathons and participate in the Iron Man is just unbelievable. Clearly, if you can get other people to think in terms of that kind discipline and perseverance, it is going to make a huge difference to them not only in their health but in everything they do.

Are there other things we can do with this program that you think would help, that would strengthen the program or encourage people to do some of the things you have done?

Ms. SEEPIE. I can only talk about my community, what they have given me, the knowledge and education about diabetes, physical fitness and eating healthy. With the SDPI, we do have a few programs like Lifestyle Balance which is a 12-week based program. It is based on nutrition, exercise and behavioral health. It gets pretty much all the components.

As an individual who was diagnosed with diabetes, I know, from feeling depression and knowing that you have diabetes at a young age, it can affect your life.

Also, I am a physical fitness specialist in my community. I teach different group exercise classes, pre-school and elementary students and seniors also. I teach a group of age groups. All I can say is, I think I am pretty much encouraging them as a regular. I think of myself as just a regular community member in my community.

When they see me, some of the kids will say, oh, you are the lady that teaches Zumba. I say, yeah, I am the lady that teaches Zumba. When can you come to Zumba class or when are you going to come to the Boys & Girls Club and teach Zumba?

I think just being a role model and encouraging people to come to our program, the Diabetes Prevention Program in Salt River is important. One good program that we have been doing is with one of our nutritionist, Maggie Fisher, is Young Wellness Warriors. I am a part of it too, as a physical fitness-exercise person. I am also in the program with my daughter.

We are educated on nutrition and also make healthy food goals in that program. They see other families in that program learning about healthy eating. We do hands-on activities. They get the chance to also help out in the kitchen cooking healthy meals. Whatever they have in the home, we provide that education and learning together as a family. I think that has helped me and some of the participants.

The CHAIRMAN. Good. I am encouraged both as I hear about your program and certainly, Mr. Eagle, about your program in terms of SDPI helping make a difference because of what you are out there doing. I appreciate it.

Senator Cortez Masto, we would turn to you at this point if you have questions.

Senator CORTEZ MASTO. Thank you, Mr. Chair, so much.

I have competing hearings going on so I have had to step in and out. But that does not mean that this topic is not important for me, particularly in the State of Nevada where we have tribal communities. I have worked with as Attorney General looking at issues affecting the health of Native communities, particularly our youth.

I have a quick question for Chairman Hawley. This whole concept of food deserts concerns me. I say that because most people do not realize in Nevada, the distance between Las Vegas and Reno is over 400 miles. That is an eight-hour drive. There is nothing but desert in between.

Just to get to an urban area, many of our tribal communities have to drive four hours with desert everywhere. I completely understand.

Can you elaborate, you may have talked about this, the food deserts and what we have done in Nevada to address this to bring healthy lifestyles but more importantly, fresh produce and fresh food to some of our communities?

Mr. HAWLEY. The concept of food deserts even in Arizona, a lot of communities, Native communities nationwide are in food deserts. A lot of our Native communities are anywhere from half a hour to four hours away from a town or what have you.

Some reservations have grocery stores on them; others do not. Some of them have local C stores. They have the local junk food and that type of thing where you go in and get your basic needs and that is about it. It is interesting that the concept exists for Natives nationwide and the access you have or do not have.

We talked about traditional resources, traditional gathering, you have hunting and fishing, all those sources but then we also will tap into the food banks where you do have the commodities. But commodities have changed over the years. The quality of the food that is provided has gotten better. Food banks have been there.

A lot of communities will refer to a town day. You have your families who will have one day out of a month designated to making those trips to town to buy everything in bulk, bring it back and store it, preserve it or freeze it. You do what you have to do. That is how you survive for the month off a town day.

You think about those things and also you consider the fact that you utilize the traditional methods of hunting and gathering. It is a real situation and it is concerning. Sitting on the panel is the first time that I have heard the term.

I started thinking about all the different things, the town days and all the planning Natives do just to go get the food you need to survive or have the nutritious meals that you count on every day, the seasonal gathering and the day-to-day activities if you are hunting or fishing, that type of thing.

I really believe that is an issue but tribes are being creative, communities are being creative. As I said, we do tap into the resources, Meals on Wheels for elders, those types of social programs that we tap into the same as any State or city taps into social service resources and human services. They are all very much a huge component of how tribes operate daily.

Senator CORTEZ MASTO. Thank you very much.

Thanks to all the panelists for being here and discussing this important topic. I do think it is an area that needs to be addressed. I think when we are talking just in general about healthy living, healthy choices, having access is the key to prevention and addressing so many of the health care issues we see in some of our tribal communities.

I appreciate all the comments today and look forward to working with all of you. Thank you again for being here.

The CHAIRMAN. Thank you, Senator.

I would turn to Vice Chairman Udall for any other questions.

Senator UDALL. Thank you.

SDPI has been flat funded for over a decade now despite the high return on investment. Admiral Buchanan and Chairman Hawley, how has the flat funding limited the impact of SDPI over the years?

Mr. BUCHANAN. The results speak for themselves. As far as the 20 years of progress we have made, the chart that was shown, activities going down to continue that process, again, it is a high priority for the agency moving forward.

Senator UDALL. When you talked about the progress going down, was that for adults and children?

Mr. BUCHANAN. That was for adults.

Senator UDALL. Adults. Is there the same number for children? Since this was authorized as a pilot program in 1997, have the numbers gone down for children?

Mr. BUCHANAN. There has not been a study that specifically focuses on children related to that for more data, but with the graph, the funding was implemented. In 1997, you can see a sharp spike coming down from that point forward.

Senator UDALL. Chairman Hawley.

Mr. HAWLEY. I can definitely say that with the flat source of funding for x amount of years, our tribal communities are growing and with the flat source of funding, I can definitely also say that. I made the statement earlier that we sometimes expect more for less. When our communities continue to grow and we have growing populations of elders and youth coming up and then you have the unborn coming up, you think about how over a year a tribe or even a community population can increase.

There is definitely an impact but the percentage, as the Admiral said, we do not know the direct impact or the percentage because we have not looked at those studies yet. Just thinking about the previous comments about doing a little bit more with a little bit less, figuratively in my mind that is what I am thinking.

We are doing a little bit more every time our populations get bigger but with the same amount of funding. How big an impact does that really have except for we are doing a little bit more work because we are addressing a larger population.

Do we have the same outputs? Possibly. We do not know. Are we doing the same thing over and over? Not likely because of the flexibility that the SDPI programs have nationwide. A lot of ideas are being implemented in different areas that are working for some areas.

Ideas are being passed back and forth. Tribes are being very creative within their programs to provide the service.

Senator UDALL. Admiral, did you have something to add on that?

Mr. BUCHANAN. I would agree that the tribes are truly the partners that are driving the innovations and changes going forward making those programs specific to their needs moving forward. That is the success behind the SDPI programs.

Senator UDALL. On the success, the numbers I have, tell me if any of you disagree with these. SDPI has supported a 61 percent growth in the use of culturally-tailored diabetes education programs which we have heard today make a real impact, if it is culturally-tailored, it is in the community and addressing the community's needs.

The CDC has linked SDPI to a 54 percent decrease in diabetes-related kidney failure in the population. Is that what was on the chart you showed us?

Mr. BUCHANAN. Yes, sir.

Senator UDALL. Thank you, Mr. Chairman.

The CHAIRMAN. I have just one follow-up question. Are you doing studies of the effect of SDPI on Native youth? You have adults and youth. Are you actually looking at the impact SDPI is having on Native youth and are you measuring that?

Mr. BUCHANAN. We are working with adults, that is what the SDPI program is designed to do, to work with the adults to reduce diabetes, since 1997. We are utilizing our programs, as mentioned earlier, related to the National Congress of American Indians. Doing specific studies right now, we are not doing that as I understand it.

The CHAIRMAN. Why?

Mr. BUCHANAN. That is a great question. We are utilizing the information we are getting from our adults. I can mention the holistic approach, going forward and utilizing those best practices as mentioned on the panel today to address our youth.

The CHAIRMAN. At this point, I would ask are there other questions from the Senators?

[No audible response.]

The CHAIRMAN. I want to turn to the panel and say to all of you, thank you very much for being here.

Members may also submit follow-up questions for the record if they so desire. The hearing record will be open for two weeks.

To all of our witnesses, thank you for the good work you are doing out there. We appreciate you being here so much.

With that, we are adjourned.

[Whereupon, at 4:20 p.m., the Committee was adjourned.]

APPENDIX

Prepared Statement of Hon. W. Ron Allen, Tribal Chairman, Jamestown S'Klallam Tribe; Board Chairman, Self-Governance Communication & Education Tribal Consortium

The Self-Governance Communication & Education Tribal Consortium1 (SGCETC), representing more than 360 Self-Governance Tribes, writes to enthusiastically endorse the success of the Special Diabetes Program for Indians (SDPI) and to support the National Indian Health Board's (NIHB) written testimony. SGCETC appreciates that the Senate Committee on Indian Affairs (SCIA) convened a hearing to highlight the success and challenges of SDPI and we submit this testimony to be included in the hearing record.

Though many issues were discussed during the hearing, SGCETC would like to provide comments and recommendations based on the proposals and priorities Self-Governance Tribes outline in the 2017–2019 Self-Governance Strategic Plan. In particular, Self-Governance Tribes would like to highlight the SDPI Diabetes Prevention Initiative's (SDPI DPI) success record and the flexibility SDPI allows for community driven solutions. We have also provided a few recommendations about how to improve the program in anticipated legislative reauthorization efforts.

Recent data illustrates SDPI is curbing the rate of Type 2 diabetes and related diseases through a lifestyle intervention program adapted from the National Institutes of Health Diabetes Prevention Program and implemented in many Tribal communities. By 2014 the structured lifestyle program showed significant improvements among participants in key behaviors and diabetes risk factors, including weight loss, BMI, healthy eating, and regular physical activity. See Table 1 below.

Overall, SDPI is producing a significant return on the federal investment and has become an effective federal initiative to combat diabetes and its complications. In Fiscal Year (FY) 2016, more than one-third of the SDPI grants and nearly forty-five percent of the total grant funds were administered by Self-Governance Tribes. SDPI has become a crucial preventative and clinical program Self-Governance Tribes use to prevent longterm illness. In fact, many Self-Governance Tribes have integrated SDPI so fully into their clinical day-to-day responsibilities it is hard to determine where one begins and the other ends. It is precisely this flexibility that has made SDPI a successful program across more than 300 unique Tribal communities.

1 The SGCETC consists of Tribal Leadership whose mission is to ensure that implementation of Tribal Self-Governance legislation and authorities in the Bureau of Indian Affairs (BIA) and Indian Health Service (IHS) are in compliance with the Tribal Self-Governance Program policies, regulations, and guidelines.

Table 1. SDPI DPI Changes in Diabetes Risk Factors

MEASURE	RESULTS	RESULTS
	Baseline 1 (n=7,097)	Follow-up 2 (n=4,549)
Weight Loss		
Mean Weight (lbs)	218	208
Mean BMI (kg/m2)	35.9	34.4
Lifestyle Behaviors		
Ate healthy foods once or more per week	77%	87%
Ate unhealthy foods less than once per week	53%	81%
Regular physical activity	30%	53%

SPDI allows Tribes to implement diabetes related programs within their clinic or as part of other health outreach programs that are separate from the physical facilities—providing access to the services no matter where the patient is located. While programs vary in their operation, each Tribe is required to identify at least one of eighteen best practices and report on the key measurements of that best practice semi-annually and annually. Additionally, SDPI grantees are required to submit to an annual Diabetes Care and Outcome audit, review the results, and adjust programs as necessary. Grantees are also required to participate in training and IHS offers free Continuing Medical Education opportunities virtually and in-person as a resource to meet that requirement. The IHS Division of Diabetes Treatment and Prevention also provides Standards of Care and Clinical Practice recommendations for clinicians to use in the treatment of patients with or at risk of developing Type 2 Diabetes—all of which are available, for anyone to access, on their website.

Self-Governance Tribes assert that the difference between maintaining the current status and decreasing rates of Type 2 Diabetes in Tribal communities largely depends on implementation of the program in the future. As such, we have a number of recommendations for Congress to consider as they plan to reauthorize the legislation prior to its expiration in September of 2017.

Permanently reauthorize SDPI. Congress established the SDPI in 1997 as part of the Balanced Budget Act to address the growing epidemic of diabetes in American Indian and Alaska Native communities. SDPI programs have become the nation's most strategic and comprehensive effort to combat diabetes. Self-Governance Tribes believe the success of these programs requires the permanent reauthorization of SDPI. We also assert that a permanent reauthorization would decrease burdensome administrative constraints SDPI grantees currently experience, such as the ability to recruit highly qualified staff on a permanent basis.

Provide a $50 million increase for SDPI. Funding for SDPI has not increased since 2001, when Congress increased support from $100 million to $150 million. An increase in funding is necessary to maintain SDPI and make a difference in the rates of Type 2 Diabetes among American Indian and Alaska Native Youth. As such, Self-Governance Tribes request that the Committee consider increasing the authorization for SDPI to $200 million. A $50 million increase will essentially level the field for SDPI grantees, as that increase only reflects inflation to 2017. As a few panelists stated, Tribes are used to doing more with less, but the time has come to provide a substantive increase that would give Tribes the room to sufficiently administer the program.

Limit oversight and administrative burden. Although improved delivery of care and increased primary prevention of Type 2 Diabetes over the past 20 years is readily documented, the annual grant application process remains cumbersome and time consuming. Tribes and Tribal Organizations are required to submit lengthy applications describing the activities and best practices on which they will report, even when the activities and funding do not significantly change. The short-term authorizations for SDPI detracts IHS and grantees from creating a long-term strategy. Self-Governance Tribes assert that, in combination with a longer or permanent authorization, longer grant periods would create more substantive change in Tribal communities, because it would encourage Tribes to track their performance over a longer period of time and set attainable goals that are based on health-related outcomes. Self-Governance Tribes also ask that a limited amount of reporting be required. Though currently data is only collected a few times a year, data collection and entry are burdensome and time consuming. The grant application process and required reporting merely result in a diversion of federal funds from their intended purpose—serving patients who have or at risk of developing Type 2 Diabetes.

Allow grantees to collect contract support costs. IHS has maintained that Tribes can only collect indirect costs related to the performance and delivery of services from within the grant award. This ultimately results in fewer services being delivered in Tribal communities. As we described above, the administrative requirements to properly implement a SDPI grant is quite burdensome. Allowing Tribes to properly account for indirect and direct costs related to the program would effectively provide grantees with an increase in funding.

SDPI continues to illustrate that healthier and stronger Tribal communities are possible with community driven, culturally applicable action plans and national best practices. As the Committee looks forward to reauthorization, we hope that you account for the flexibility needed to properly implement a prevention and treatment program in Tribal communities across the country and consider the positive effects a long-term reauthorization, funding increase, and simplification of oversight could have in the success of SDPI.

In closing, SGCETC would like to thank the Committee for the opportunity to submit testimony. We look forward to working with you on the successful SDPI reauthorization.

PREPARED STATEMENT OF ALLISON BARLOW, PH.D, MA, MPH, DIRECTOR, CENTER FOR AMERICAN INDIAN HEALTH, JOHNS HOPKINS BLOOMBERG SCHOOL OF PUBLIC HEALTH

Dear Senators Hoeven and Udall,

I am writing as Director of the Center for American Indian Health at the Johns Hopkins Bloomberg School of Public Health, to request that my written testimony be included in the record for the hearing on March 29, 2017 entitled "Native Youth: Promoting Diabetes Prevention through Healthy Living." In my expert opinion, the Special Diabetes Prevention Initiative (SPDI) has produced very positive results and I urge you to encourage your colleagues to consider level funding at $150 million in the FY17 and FY18 budgets.

Congress's continued support for SPDI will yield tremendous return on investment by hastening the discovery of cost-effective solutions for preventing diabetes for all Americans through a proven program that has demonstrated sound evidence and accountability.

The Johns Hopkins Center for American Indian Health has held a Memorandum of Understanding with Indian Health Service (IHS) since its founding in 1991. Johns Hopkins and IHS leverage research findings and disseminate best practices to overcome tribal health disparities. The Center also works to scale up solutions found effective with American Indian communities to other vulnerable American communities.

In terms of of public health impact, my colleagues and I at the Johns Hopkins Center for American Indian Health cannot overstate the importance of the 1997-enacted SPDI to American Indian and Alaska Native health and well-being. The achievements that have occurred over the past 20 years are of tremendous public health significance: these achievements include a decrease in type 2 diabetes in American Indian and Alaska Native youth, a 54 percent reduction in end-stage renal disease between 1997–2013, and the levelling off of obesity levels in American Indian children.

This progress has occurred through congressionally-appropriated resources ($150 million/year) that Indian Health Service has been able to extend to 301 tribal communities across 35 states. Through the leadership of the IHS Diabetes Program director, Ann Bullock, MD, these dollars have materialized into comprehensive, creative, and effective prevention strategies that are now being recognized as a model for the nation and the world. For example, a leading international journal just published a reference to SPDI impact:

> A promising new report demonstrates a substantial decline in the incidence of diabetic end-stage renal disease among American Indians and Alaska Natives, coinciding with a public health intervention targeting diabetes management in this population. This success may offer a model for interventions to improve kidney disease outcomes in other high-risk populations.—*C. Wyatt, Kidney International* (2017) 91, 766–768

However, the work of SPDI is not done. American Indian and Alaska Native children and families still shoulder the greatest disparities in obesity, diabetes, and related health and workforce consequences of any racial or ethnic group in the nation. This constellation of disease is the result of forced lifestyle changes brought about through colonization. The degradation of American Indian health due to commercialized diets and sedentary lifestyles forecasts what will be the fate of the majority of Americans if we don't continue to discover effective public health intervention to curb obesity and diabetes. Further, building interventions with the highest risk, lowest-income population makes the most scientific and economic sense.

Sustained investment in SPDI will continue to produce fruitful innovations for high-risk populations and ultimately save our nation inestimable costs in human suffering, lost productivity, and health care and workforce dollars. Indeed, Dr. Bullock's latest work through SPDI to support intervention with expectant parents through children's early life (0 to 3 years) is designed to prevent diabetes starting in the womb. Early life intervention could revolutionize how we will protect children's health and our nation's prosperity.

Thank you for including these comments in the record.

PREPARED STATEMENT OF UNITED SOUTH AND EASTERN TRIBES SOVEREIGNTY PROTECTION FUND (USET SPF)

United South and Eastern Tribes Sovereignty Protection Fund (USET SPF) is pleased to provide the Senate Committee on Indian Affairs (SCIA) with testimony for the record of its March 29th oversight hearing, "Native Youth: Promoting Diabetes Prevention Through Healthy Living." USET SPF appreciates the SCIA for making the reauthorization of the Special Diabetes Program for Indians (SDPI) a priority for this Congress. The SDPI program has made inroads in diabetes care and prevention in Indian Country, including in the development of youth education and prevention initiatives. The program must be reauthorized this Fiscal Year.

USET SPF is a non-profit, inter-tribal organization representing 26 federally recognized Tribal Nations from Texas across to Florida and up to Maine.[1] USET SPF is dedicated to enhancing the development of federally recognized Indian Tribal Nations, to improving the capabilities of Tribal governments, and assisting USET SPF Member Tribal Nations in dealing effectively with public policy issues and in serving the broad needs of Indian people. This includes advocating for the full exercise of inherent Tribal sovereignty.

Special Diabetes Program for Indians (SDPI) and Diabetes Prevention Programs

In response to the disproportionately high rate of type 2 diabetes in American Indians and Alaska Native (AI/AN) communities, Congress passed the Balanced Budget Act in 1997 establishing the SDPI as a grant program for the prevention and treatment of diabetes at a funding level of $30 million per year for five years. After extensive Tribal consultation, the Indian Health Service (IHS) distributed the funding to over 300 IHS, Tribal and Urban AI/AN health programs. In 2001, Congress increased the amount of SDPI funding to $100 million per year, and then again increased it to $150 million per year from 2004–2010, which was then extended for an additional 3 years through Fiscal Year (FY) 2013. Since FY 2013, SDPI had been extended in one year increments, however, the most recent extension as a part of the 'Doc Fix' legislation in June of 2015, authorized two additional years at $150 million/year through September 30, 2017. With SDPI set to expire this year, it is critical that this Congress prioritize its reauthorization.

In the Indian Health Service (IHS) Nashville Area, the prevalence rate of diabetes is 23 percent, which is 3.6 times higher than the U.S. all races age-adjusted rate of 6.4 percent. Rates can be even higher in individual USET SPF states, like Louisiana and Mississippi, where prevalence rates for our member Tribal Nations are at 29.5 percent and 36.7 percent, respectively. Despite the severity of the epidemic, Tribal Nations have implemented successful and culturally relevant diabetes prevention and treatment activities through the SDPI grant program.

USET[2] has been an SDPI grantee since its inception, and is unique in that it applies for the SDPI grant on behalf of 20 of its member Tribal Nations as the primary grantee. USET then enters into subcontract agreements with participating Tribal Nations for local program implementation. Our member Tribal Nations continue to feel this is the easiest and best grant option for them, as many are small communities with limited staffing and resources to write a grant of this magnitude. USET's administration of grant dollars allows local level staff to focus on the prevention, care, and treatment of diabetes within their communities.

Through SDPI and its Diabetes Prevention Program (DP, a program piloted as part of the larger SDPI), Tribal Nations have built significant infrastructure to address the health needs of their pre-diabetic and diabetic citizens. This includes diabetes specific health providers, regular testing and monitoring, nutritionists, fitness programs, and patient education. In addition to avoiding the more costly consequences of diabetes, like End Stage Renal Disease and limb amputations, among the diabetic population, Tribal SDPI programs have successfully prevented the disease among at-risk groups. In fact, after steadily increasing over the preceding two decades, between 2000 and 2011, incidence rates of ESRD in AI/AN people with diabetes decreased 43 percent—more than for any other racial group in the U.S.[3]

---

[1] USET SPF member Tribal Nations include: Alabama-Coushatta Tribe of Texas (TX), Aroostook Band of Micmac Indians (ME), Catawba Indian Nation (SC), Cayuga Nation (NY), Chitimacha Tribe of Louisiana (LA), Coushatta Tribe of Louisiana (LA), Eastern Band of Cherokee Indians (NC), Houlton Band of Maliseet Indians (ME), Jena Band of Choctaw Indians (LA), Mashantucket Pequot Indian Tribe (CT), Mashpee Wampanoag Tribe (MA), Miccosukee Tribe of Indians of Florida (FL), Mississippi Band of Choctaw Indians (MS), Mohegan Tribe of Indians of Connecticut (CT), Narragansett Indian Tribe (RI), Oneida Indian Nation (NY), Passamaquoddy Tribe at Indian Township (ME), Passamaquoddy Tribe at Pleasant Point (ME), Penobscot Indian Nation (ME), Poarch Band of Creek Indians (AL), Saint Regis Mohawk Tribe (NY), Seminole Tribe of Florida (FL), Seneca Nation of Indians (NY), Shinnecock Indian Nation (NY), Tunica-Biloxi Tribe of Louisiana (LA), and the Wampanoag Tribe of Gay Head (Aquinnah) (MA).

[2] USET, or United South and Eastern Tribes, is the 501(c)3 sister organization to USET SPF, which is a 501(c)4. USET provides programmatic and technical support to our 26 member Tribal Nations.

[3] IHS SDPI 2014 Report to Congress.

In 2004, through the SDPI program, IHS piloted the DP program to implement lifestyle interventions, which were found effective through clinical trials in the National Institutes of Health-led clinical trial on diabetes prevention throughout the federal system. By May 2014, approximately 4,549 high-risk AI/AN participants completed program courses on healthy lifestyle interventions. Among those that completed the program, 87 percent of participants ate healthy foods once or more per week versus the pre-intervention baseline of 77 percent and 53 percent engaged regularly in physical activity compared to 30 percent pre-intervention. IHS estimates that the incidence rate of diabetes for participants in the SDPI DP was 6.5 percent compared to the 11 percent for the NIH Placebo group. The lower rates of diabetes incidence show the efficacy of SDPI DP interventions and the success of diabetes prevention infrastructure in Indian Country.

Challenges with Diabetes Prevention Program Certifications

Although we acknowledge the importance of evidence-based Diabetes Prevention Programs (DPP) through the Centers for Disease Control and Prevention (CDC), we do not believe this is the only approach for Indian Country in administering quality prevention programs. This is because many USET SPF member Tribal Nations do not have the capacity to meet the strict eligibility criteria and program requirements. USET SPF is currently aware of at least one Tribal Nation health program with CDC DPP certification at risk of losing its certification due to on-going challenges with recruitment of patients meeting the eligibility criteria, as well as overly narrow quality and reimbursement indicators. These indicators have unrealistic target thresholds and should be subject to individual targets that better meet the health objectives of a particular program. Additionally, the current criteria omits indicators on behavioral change, which are important for measuring the success of these lifestyle interventions. Indicators should include behavioral change measures related to diet and exercise, which are major factors in diabetes prevention and were proven effective through the SDPI DP pilot. In order for our Tribal Nations to continue programming with CDC DPP certification, these flexibilities are necessary to account for the unique circumstances and challenges of diabetes prevention work in Indian Country.

Similar challenges exist for our smaller member Tribal Nations which operate SDPI programs and may wish to seek CDC DPP certification in the future. Under the current criteria, many USET SPF member Tribal Nations would be precluded from participation due to a lack of capacity, staffing shortages, and small populations of patients meeting patient eligibility criteria. Many of these Nations do not have the staffing bandwidth to undertake the administrative burdens of applying for CDC DPP or American Diabetes Association recognition.

SDPI Advancements

Like other Tribal Nations across the country, USET SPF Tribal Nations suffer disproportionately from a variety of health issues, leading oftentimes to a severely reduced quality of life and life span. AI/ANs suffer from obesity, hypertension, heart disease, and diabetes at rates much higher than the general U.S. population. Data shows that AI/ANs have the highest rates of diabetes in the U.S. and are more than twice as likely as white adults to have diabetes. IHS' SDPI grant program is beginning to turn these statistics around. Recent data shows that through SDPI, USET Tribal Nations have made significant progress. Between 2013 and 2015, USET Tribal Nations increased the percentage of:

- Healthy blood sugar in our diabetes patients from 45 percent to 49 percent;
- Normal blood pressure from 60 percent to 62 percent; and
- The rate of annual eye exams from 45 percent to 55 percent.

Through collaborations, best practices, and prevention initiatives resulting from SDPI, our Tribal Nations are making strides. Nashville Area AI/ANs are living longer with diabetes, with increased access to specialty care and better control of the disease, all due to this essential program.

For example, the Passamaquoddy Tribe of Maine (USET SDPI sub contractor) is working in partnership with the University of Maine's Cooperative Extension Program and the Pleasant Point Health Center SDPI Program collaborated on two community programs, the first being a 4-week program called Dining with Diabetes Down East. The program was adapted to include information specific to the Passamaquoddy community, culturally specific foods, and some use of the Passamaquoddy language. Each session included a presentation, cooking demonstrations, and facilitated discussion. An overview of the Diabetes "ABCs" (A1C, Blood Pleasure and Cholesterol) was presented during the first session and the other sessions covered other aspects of diabetes prevention. The program gave many participants a new outlook on traditional foods and culture within their communities, while developing healthy habits for long-term prevention.

The second program was teaching the Diabetes Education in Tribal Schools (DETS) curriculum to pre-school, kindergarten, first, and second grade students from October 2015—March 2016. The children and teachers learned about more and less healthy foods and activities; and about diabetes. One of the last classes involved bringing in a community member with diabetes so that the students could ask them questions about the disease. The success of the program is due to the collaborative effort between the teachers, students, Pleasant Point Health Center SDPI program and the University of Maine Cooperative Extension. These collaborations are only some of the impacts that SDPI has had on Tribal communities, including youth.

Native Youth: Obesity and Diabetes Rates

The impacts of obesity and diabetes on Native youth are troubling. In the IHS Nashville Area, Tribal Nations have been able to maintain the low rates of diabetes for youth under 20 years of age (accounting for less than 1 percent of the total diabetes population) within our communities. However, many USET SPF Tribal Nation battle high youth obesity rates, with over half of the youth between the ages of 2 and 5 years falling into the obese body mass index ranges. Some initiatives that USET SPF Tribal Nations are utilizing through SDPI to decrease these rates are:

- Teaching the DETS curriculum in schools or after school programs;
- Making healthy food choices available and fun/interesting to Native youth;
- Learning about traditional Tribal Nation foods and incorporating them into diets;
- Providing healthier foods in vending machines;
- Providing healthy cooking and/or snack preparation classes for kids; and
- Limiting fast food meals for kids and providing quick, easy, healthy options for families on the go.

SDPI plays an important role in ensuring USET SPF Tribal Nations are able to reduce high rates of obesity among our youth. These types of interventions reduce the incidence of risk factors for diabetes, such as obesity, providing long-term health benefits.

Access to Healthy Food and Fresh Vegetables

Tribal Nations are located in some of the most rural and impoverished communities, lacking overall access to health care and healthy food options. Limited access to healthier foods, such as fresh vegetables, is often times a barrier to maintaining a healthy diet. USET SPF member Tribal Nations vary in their ability access to healthier food options, but through SDPI, all are utilizing methods to increase traditional foods and healthier options available to Tribal communities. SDPI has allowed for community and school gardens, providing access to healthier and fresh foods, while encouraging physical activity. Tribal Nations are incorporating traditional foods and language into these gardens as a means to maintaining community and youth cultural knowledge and the foods our ancestors consumed.

Reauthorize SDPI

Despite its documented success, funding for SDPI has been flat since 2004, even as inflation and medical costs rise. Tribal Nations and Congress have made significant investments in preventing and managing diabetes. In order to continue making progress in the fight against the disease in Indian Country, SDPI must be reauthorized this Fiscal Year to avoid the loss of Tribal programs, prevention, and progress. Any lapse in reauthorization will cause the costs of diabetes and its complications to increase again for Tribal communities, and precious jobs created by this program will cease. USET SPF is urging Congress to reauthorize the SDPI for multiple years at no less $150 million/year, with incremental increases each year based on medical inflation rates. Congress must not allow this successful investment to lapse, just as its effects arebeing realized in the form of strong data and widespread lifestyle changes. Timely reauthorization will ensure that Tribal Nations can continue the fight against this epidemic without interruption.

Conclusion

USET SPF appreciates the opportunity to provide comments following the SCIA hearing on Native Youth: Promoting Diabetes Prevention through Healthy Living. Over the past 19 years, Indian Country has been leading the fight against the diabetes epidemic, and assisting patients and communities affected by the disease. Congress and IHS, along with Tribal Nations, recognize the importance and effectiveness of SDPI interventions in improving and maintaining the health of Tribal communities. USET SPF urges this Congress to reauthorize SDPI before it expires on September 30, 2017, and looks forward to working with the Committee on advancing this vital legislation.

———

PREPARED STATEMENT OF KAMANA'OPONO M. CRABBE, PH.D. (KA POUHANA)/CEO, OFFICE OF HAWAIIAN AFFAIRS (OHA)

Aloha e Honorable Chairman John Hoeven, Vice Chairman Tom Udall, and members of the Senate Committee on Indian Affairs,

Mahalo (thank you) for the opportunity to submit testimony regarding the Committee's March 29, 201 7 Oversight Hearing on "Native Youth: Promoting Diabetes Prevention Through Healthy Living." The Office of Hawaiian Affairs (OHA) is a public trust and independent state agency established through the Hawai'i State Constitution to improve the lives of Hawai'i's indigenous people (Native Hawaiians). OHA's enabling statute charges it to advocate on behalf of Native Hawaiians, and to assess policies and practices as they may affect Native Hawaiians. OHA is also named in various federal statutes as a recognized Native Hawaiian organization with standing to be consulted with on matters pertaining to Native Hawaiian rights and cultural resources. With that kuleana (responsibility) in mind, our agency is pleased to submit testimony for the record.

OHA operates under a strategy plan which includes Mauli OIa (health) as a strategic priority of the agency. Our agency collaborates with various organizations to strengthen our community's resources in six strategic priorities, including health. We employ the Native Hawaiian framework of Mauli Ola in our work to advance the health and well-being of Native Hawaiians. In this framework, individual health is connected to a number of environmental and social factors, also known as social determinants of health. We focus on physical, emotional, mental, and spiritual health, as well as social, economic, and environmental factors influencing health and wellbeing at each stage of our beneficiaries' lives. Ancestral wisdom as well as mainstream historical record and scientific research reflects that prior to regular Western contact, Native Hawaiians were a thriving, abundantly healthy people living in what Congress, through Public Law 103–1 50 described as "a highly organized, self-sufficient, subsistent social system based on communal land tenure with a sophisticated language, culture, and religion."

Unfortunately, Western contact and the erosion of Native Hawaiian control over our resources greatly disrupted the land-based social determinants of health that Native Hawaiians had established. Since then, the health challenges laced by the Native Hawaiian community have greatly evolved. While communicable diseases were once the greatest threat facing the Native Hawaiian community in the late eighteenth through early twentieth century, noncommunicable diseases pose a serious threat today. In this respect and others, we share many of the needs and concerns of our American Indian and Alaska Native brothers and sisters. Many chronic diseases, especially asthma, hypertension, and diabetes, have a higher prevalence within the Native Hawaiian community in comparison with the general population of the State of Hawai'i.[1] It has been estimated that one in three Native Hawaiian adults have or are at-risk for diabetes or pre-diabetes.[2] In 2010, the age-adjusted prevalence rate of Native Hawaiians living with diabetes was 84.4 per 1,000 people, while the State of Hawai'i's overall prevalence was 59.9 per 1,000 people.[3]

According to the Centers for Disease Control and Prevention (CDC), there are a number of risk factors that increase the likelihood of developing diabetes. Obesity is one such factor strongly linked with the development of Type 2 Diabetes.[4] Pa-

---

[1] See OFFICE OF HAWAIIAN AFFAIRS, NATIVE HAWAIIAN HEALTH FACT SHEET 2015, VOL.1, CHRONIC DISEASE, available at *http://i19of32x2y133s8o4xzaOgf14.wpengine.netdna-cdn.com/wp-content/uploads/Volume-1-Chronic-Diseases-FINAL.pdf.*

[2] 2See UNIVERSITY OF HAWAI'I AT MANOA JOHN A. BURNS SCHOOL OF MEDICINE CENTER FOR NATIVE AND PACIFIC HEALTH DISPARITIES RESEARCH DEPARTMENT OF NATIVE HAWAIIAN HEALTH, ASSESSMENT AND PRIORITIES FOR HEALTH & WELL–BEING IN NATIVE HAWAIIANS & OTHER PACIFIC PEOPLES, available at *http://www.hicore.org/media/assets/JABSOMStudyreNHHealth_20131.pdf*

[3] 3See OFFICE OF HAWAIIAN AFFAIRS, NATIVE HAWAIIAN HEALTH FACT SHEET 2015, VOL.1, CHRONIC DISEASE, available at *http://19of32x2y133s8o4xzaOgIl4.wpengine.netdna-cdn.com/wp-content/uploads/Volume-1-Chronic-Diseases-FINAL.pdf*

[4] See CENTERS FOR DISEASE CONTROL AND PREVENTION, NATIONAL CENTER FOR CHRONIC DISEASE PREVENTION AND HEALTH PROMOTION, DIABETES REPORT CARD 2014, available at *https://www.cdc.gov/diabetes/pdfs/library/diabetesreportcard2014.pdf*

tients who are obese and diagnosed with Type 2 Diabetes often have poor control of their blood sugar, blood pressure, and cholesterol, which can all lead to severe health complications.[5] Obesity is a problem facing the Native Hawaiian community. In 201 2, the Native Hawaiian obesity rate in Hawai'i was 44 4%[6] This rate is in stark contrast to the State of HawaVi's relatively low obesity rate of 23.6 percent, which is much lower than most of the nation.[7] Native Hawaiian youth are also affected by obesity, and Native Hawaiian public school students have a rate that is much higher than their peers in the State.[8]

OHA currently funds a number of programs in Hawai'i that use the Mauli Ola framework for diabetes treatment and prevention for Native Hawaiians. One such program, the Hua Ola Project, is managed by the Boys & Girls Club of the Big Island, and instills lifelong fitness and dietary habits in youth through culturally responsive experiential education. Another program currently funded by OHA is I Ola Lahui's KUlana Hawai'i project, which provides comprehensive, culturally-minded weight and chronic disease management services to Native Hawaiian adults and their families. The continued delivery of innovative programs that focus on Native Hawaiian adults and emphasize youth education is critical to addressing the health disparities of Native Hawaiians. Beyond these critical initiatives, Papa OIa Lokahi and the five Native Hawaiian Health Care Systems located within the State provide research, education, and other services, as well as foster and encourage collaborations for a holistic approach to health care in the Native Hawaiian community broadly.

Significant health improvements have been achieved in programs integrating cultural practices into health interventions.[9] To create a lasting effect on the health of Native Hawaiians and decrease diabetes prevalence in the Native Hawaiian community, Native Hawaiian adults, youth, and families must be provided the opportunity to engage in these types of healthy living programs, diabetes management education, and other diabetes prevention programs and culturally-grounded services in the Mauli Ola framework.

OHA once again thanks the Committee for holding this oversight hearing on Native youth and the promotion of healthy lifestyles. This important topic needs to continue to be addressed in Native American, Alaska Native, and Native Hawaiian communities. We humbly ask that Hawai'i's indigenous people also be considered in whatever legislative and oversight initiatives Congress engages in to address these important issues. I look forward to continuing to work with you on these issues and others affecting our Native people.

PREPARED STATEMENT OF PATRICK M. ROCK, MD, CEO, INDIAN HEALTH BOARD OF MINNEAPOLIS, INC.

Dear Senator:

On behalf of the Indian Health Board of Minneapolis, I thank you for your interest in the issues that are important to American Indian/Alaska Native (AI/AN) people. My clinic is also a proud member of the National Council of Urban Indian Health, which represents the interests of the more than 40 urban Indian health providers (UIHPs) the Congress has established in far-flung locations across the nation to serve urban Indians, who constitute more than 70 percent of all AI/AN people.

AI/AN adults are 2.3 times more likely to have diabetes compared with non-Hispanic whites and the death rate due to diabetes for AI/AN is 1.6 times higher than the general U.S. population. SDPI, which is an indispensable part of the solution to this scourge, supports over 330 diabetes treatment and prevention programs in 35 states, which have led to significant advances in diabetes education, prevention, and treatment.

The good news is SDPI works and it saves money in the long run. In 2000–2011, the incidence rate of End-Stage Renal Disease (ESRD) in AI/AN people with diabe-

---

[5] *Ibid.*

[6] See OFFICE OF HAWAIIAN AFFAIRS, NATIVE HAWAIIAN HEALTH FACT SHEET 2015, VOL.1, CHRONIC DISEASE, available at *http://19of32x2yl33s8o4xzaOgf14.wpengine.netdna-cdn.com/wp-content/uploads/Volume-l-Chronic-Diseases-FINAL.pdf*

[7] *Ibid.*

[8] *Ibid.*

[9] 9See UNIVERSITY OF HAWAI'I AT MANOA JOHN A. BURNS SCHOOL OF MEDICINE CENTER FOR NATIVE AND PACIFIC HEALTH DISPARITIES RESEARCH DEPARTMENT OF NATIVE HAWAIIAN HEALTH, ASSESSMENT AND PRIORITIES FOR HEALTH & WELL–BEING IN NATIVE HAWAIIANS & OTHER PACIFIC PEOPLES, available at *http://www.hicore.org/media/assets/JABSOMStudyreNH__Health__20131.pdf*

tes declined by 43 percent—a greater decline than any other racial or ethnic group. ESRD is the largest cost-driver of Medicare costs.

Reduction in the incidence rate translates into significant cost savings for Medicare, the IHS, and third party payers.

S. 747 would reauthorize SDPI for seven years—from fiscal year 2018 through fiscal year 2024—at no increase in cost other than taking into account health care inflation. I urge you to cosponsor The Special Diabetes Program for Indians Reauthorization Act of 2017 (S. 747), which was recently introduced by Senator Tom Udall (D–NM). SDPI will be shut down on September 30 if the program is not reauthorized in time. If SDPI's reauthorization is not to fall through the cracks, it is imperative that Senator Udall's bill be supported through co-sponsorships.

SDPI has become the most comprehensive treatment and prevention programing available to NA/AI in the Minneapolis-St Paul Metro area. We are one of the longest funded programs in the United States. We have also been recognized nationally and locally in providing innovative diabetes programing.

Thanks for your consideration of my views. Please let me know if you will cosponsor S. 747, so I can share the news with our clinic's patients and providers. I will check in with your staff in two weeks on this matter because so much is at stake for Indian Country. Please let me know if you have any questions.

PREPARED STATEMENT OF ASHLEY TUOMI, PRESIDENT, NATIONAL COUNCIL OF URBAN INDIAN HEALTH

On behalf of the National Council of Urban Indian Health (NCUIH), which represents urban Indian health care programs (UIHPs) across the nation that provide high-quality, culturally-competent care to urban Indians, who constitute more than 70 percent of all American Indians/Alaska Natives (AI/AN), I, Ashley Tuomi, NCUIH's President, submit this testimony for the record in relation to the March 29, 2017, oversight hearing held by the Senate Committee on Indian Affairs on the Special Diabetes Program for Indians (SDPI).

I thank Chairman Hoeven for holding this hearing as well as his interest in SDPI and Ranking Member Udall for his recent introduction of the Special Diabetes Program for Indians Reauthorization Act of 2017 (S. 747), which NCUIH strongly supports. S. 747 would reauthorize SDPI for seven years-from fiscal year 2018 through fiscal year 2024—at no increase in cost other than taking into account health care inflation. NCUIH urges Senators to cosponsor this important legislation in order to show the support necessary to secure SDPI's timely reauthorization.

It is imperative that SDPI be reauthorized before its expiration on September 30. Grants to health care providers in Indian Country made pursuant to SDPI have been instrumental in the marked reduction in the incidence rate of diabetes-and the related savings to Medicare, the Indian Health Service (IHS), and third party providers.

At NCUIH's recent Washington Summit, timely reauthorization of SDPI was one of our organization's top legislative priorities, even with a broad and comprehensive legislative agenda. The failure to reauthorize this program would severely undermine the promising progress UIHPs and Indian Country have made against diabetes. UIHPs are proud of their role in the fight against diabetes,—Out of the 301 SDPI grants, 30 grants (out of 43 urban programs) went to UIHPs, or 6.65 percent of the $136,074,763 SDPI funds awarded nationally.

The Committee is very familiar with the grim statistics of the toll that diabetes inflicts on Indian Country. AI/AN adults are 2.3 times more likely to have diabetes compared with non-Hispanic whites and the death rate due to diabetes for AI/AN is 1.6 times higher than the general U.S. population. And the costs in dollars are also extraordinary—in 2012 alone 11 percent of AI/AN with diabetes accounted for 37 percent of all IHS adult treatment costs.

However, the Committee also knows that SDPI achieves outstanding results and that the program saves significant money in the long run. SDPI supports over 330 diabetes treatment and prevention programs in 35 states, which have led to significant advances in diabetes education, prevention, and treatment. In 2000–2011, the incidence rate of End-Stage Renal Disease (ESRD) in AI/AN people with diabetes declined by 43%—a greater decline than any other racial or ethnic group. ESRD is the largest cost-driver of Medicare costs. Reduction in the incidence rate translates into significant cost savings for Medicare, third party payers, as well as IHS.

Let me tell the Committee how seven UIHPs have used SDPI funds to provide valuable services which have transformed and saved their patients' lives.

First, we can start in the northeast to Detroit, Michigan where my own program, *American Indian Health and Family Services,* resides. Last year we attempted to refer clients for services outside of the agency that we sponsored with SDPI funds for diabetic testing, but we found that program unsuccessful, as patients were unlikely to follow-up with the referral. During this fiscal year we changed course and decided with SDPI funds we would purchase a retinal camera that now allows us to do undialated eye exams in the clinic. Now that we have our own equipment in house, we are able to catch the patients right when they enter our facility and there has been an immediately increase in retinal eye exams. We are catching diabetes as soon as it enters the door, thanks to SDPI funding.

Then we can travel to the Great Plains, at the *South Dakota Urban Indian Health (SDUIH)*, which serves both Pierre and Sioux Falls with full-time primary and behavioral health clinics.

SDUIH has participated in the SDPI program for fifteen years. Throughout this time, SDUIH, with its accreditation from the American Diabetes Association, has provided direct diabetes patient education, prevention and treatment services that benefits those who have diabetes as well as those who are at high-risk of getting diabetes.

SDPI funds have made it possible for SDUIH to add physical fitness centers located on-site within the clinic facility that offer new and state-of-the-art equipment. SDUIH has also added a fully operational teaching kitchen that allows patients to participate in cooking classes and learn how to improve their diets.

SDPI funds support the program's grocery store tours during which patients are accompanied by a care manager who teaches them how to shop for healthier and more nutritious food. Funds have also been used to purchase the lab equipment necessary for operating a high-level diabetes program, including Piccolo machines, DCA Vantage Analyzers, and HemoCue testing devices.

SDPI funds allow SDUIH to employ highly-qualified staff to prevent and treat diabetes, including certified educators, registered dieticians, licensed nutritionists, fitness/yoga class instructors, and child care providers.

Ms. Donna LC Keeler, the SDUIH Executive Director, reports that SDPI funds have allowed her program to provide a wide array of services to the diabetic patients serviced by SDUIH. According to the most recent Indian Health Service Annual Diabetes Audit, 59 percent of the program's patients have had diabetes less than 20 years and 79 percent are diagnosed with comorbidity of hypertension which demonstrates the need of continued funding and services. Positive results from SDPI for the SDUIH program include 55 percent of their patients having blood sugar (A1c) control of 7.9 or less and 77 percent having blood pressure of 140/90 or less, so progress is being made but there still is so much left to do.

Thanks to SDUIH's use of SDPI funds, 100 percent of all diabetic patients are screened for tobacco use; 97 percent have comprehensive foot exams; 77 percent have retinal imaging eye exams; 71 percent have annual dental exams; 99 percent have diabetes education; 97 percent have physical activity education; 85 percent have flu/pneumococcal vaccines; 73 percent have hepatitis B immunizations; and 100 percent of diabetic patients are screened for depression.

Ms. Keeler sums up the fight being waged by SDUIH against diabetes: "While, clearly, SDPI has been a success—lives of patients have been saved and their health status has been improved—much work remains to be done. Without SDPI funds, SDUIH would not be able to retain the dedicated diabetes staff that have accomplished so much for so many patients. It is critical to continue funding in order to fight against diabetes in Indian County."

Let's shift our focus to Tulsa, Oklahoma, where the Indian community is served by the *Indian Health Care Resource Center of Tulsa (IHCRC)*, a comprehensive clinic which cares for almost 12,000 patients annually. Accredited by the American Association of Diabetes Educators, IHCRC has used SDPI funds for almost 20 years to offer a variety of programming, including diabetes case management, fitness and exercise, nutrition counseling, and diabetes education.

Ms. Carmelita Skeeter, the program's chief executive officer, reports that during FY2016 alone, IHCRC's diabetes program served 1,410 duplicated patients in the clinic for diabetes case management (63), diabetes education (649), diet management (604), and exercise/fitness education (94). Specific program goals include glycemic control, nutrition education, and physical activity education. IHCRC's public health nurse, originally funded through the Healthy Heart program and now through SDPI, coordinates community efforts and the integration of diabetes case management into primary care, especially for repeatedly non-compliant patients.

A chart audit of 881 patients with diabetes revealed that 77 percent had known hypertension and 72 percent had a Body Mass Index (BMI) of 30.00 or above (obesity). Based on BMI, one-third of IHCRC's 3,700 patients under the age of 18 are overweight or obese. With this information in mind, IHCRC knows that helping patients to develop a healthy lifestyle can also help to end the vicious cycle of this disease.

IHCRC's diabetes programs have been enhanced in recent years to include prevention, especially for youth and families. Collaboration with the N7 Fund, Southern Plains Tribal Health Board, and an area funder have helped to further expand the programs.

Programs range from summer wellness camps to training teachers and youth workers to use physical activity in teaching. This teaching style has proven to activate the brain, improve on-task behavior during academic instruction time, and increase daily physical activity levels among children. The *Sit Less, Move More, Learn Better* program, attended by approximately 60 teachers and youth workers each year, has helped more than 70,000 youth across Oklahoma.

The youth fitness and diabetes prevention program includes *Summer Wellness Camp*, a youth run club (initially funded by the N7 Fund), youth fitness programs, and two annual *Family, Fun and Fitness Days*. Each year, more than 300 youth attend the camp which focuses on diabetes prevention, healthy lifestyles, leadership, team-building, cultural experiences, and problem-solving.

The annual family fun and fitness festival, attended by more than 450 people since inception, brings families together in an active environment. The day's highlight is the *One Mile Fun Run and Walk*.

The program's fight against diabetes has been further enhanced by engaging youth and families in a running club in which 25 youth and their family members participate. The club meets every Saturday morning to run together and participates in approximately six community runs during the year. During the winter group members work out at the YMCA and participate as a club in social activities and community service.

"No one could have ever anticipated the changes that occurred in the running club participants," reports Ms. Skeeter. "Youth have become stronger and healthier. They have become socially connected with one another and with others they have met through community races. Families have begun running and working out together. Youth self-esteem has improved. Youth have learned to provide encouragement to others including their own family members. Community volunteers including members of American Electric Power's Native American employee group have become extremely involved with the club. Overall, the diabetes education program has made significant strides in diabetes prevention for youth and families."

Like Ms. Keeler, her counterpart in South Dakota, Ms. Skeeter is a passionate supporter of SDPI, having seen modest amounts of money turn around the lives of so many Tulsans in such meaningful ways, and she is also determined to see the program reauthorized.

Let's take the I–44 west and learn how the *Oklahoma City Indian Clinic (OKCIC)* has used SDPI funds for 18 years to provide essential services to its 2,948 patients with diabetes, 2,994 patients with prediabetes, and 4,672 youth patients, out of an active patient clinic population of 18,077.

Beginning in 2001, reports Ms. Robyn Sunday-Allen, OKCIC's chief executive officer, SDPI funds began paying for the program's first *Teaching Urbans Roads To Lifestyle & Exercise (TURTLE) Camp* for children. This initial day camp for OKCIC youth was focused on diabetes prevention for children 12 to 16 years of age. Sessions on nutrition, exercise, diabetes education, drug and alcohol abuse, tobacco abuse have been held by OKCIC for the past 16 years.

SDPI funding has also allowed OKCIC to add a wellness center to the clinic's campus. Patients are able to work out individually, participate in group activities or meet with a personal trainer/life coach. In fact, the wellness center has become the social community for OKCIC patients as they participate in group fitness classes, diabetes prevention/education meetings, cooking classes, and cultural activities.

Recognizing the importance of good nutrition, OKCIC began holding cooking demonstration classes in 2013, and SDPI funding helped to equip a kitchen. All patients and their families are welcome to learn from the registered dietitian/chef to see how to prepare healthy foods within a reasonable budget. Participation in the cooking classes has increased from 560 visits in 2013 to 1670 in 2016.

In addition, OKCIC provides annual back-to-school physicals, immunizations and screening at the program's *Children's Health Fair*. Through these screenings, youth at risk are referred to follow-up services where parents and their children receive education to make the necessary changes to develop healthy lifestyle habits. "SDPI funding," reports Ms. Sunday-Allen, "allows OKCIC to go beyond being simply an ambulatory health care facility, which helps to endow our patients with the courage to move towards healthier lifestyles."

OKCIC, thanks in large part to SDPI funds, provides disease prevention programming to AI/AN children in an effort to prevent Type 2 diabetes and related comorbidities. These programs include weekly afterschool programs, school break programs and 1:1 nutrition and physical activity counseling. Afterschool programming includes boxing, adventure sports, running, golf, and tennis. School break programs include, in addition to *TURTLE Camp: Kids in the Kitchen*, swimming lessons, *NYPD Camp (Native Youth Preventing Diabetes)*, jump rope camp, basketball camp, dance clinic, culture camp and *NKOG Camp (Native Kids on the Go!)*.

All interventions assess children for weight status, acanthosis nigricans, blood pressure and obesity-causing behaviors such as sugar-sweetened beverage intake, fruit and vegetable intake, physical activity engagement and screen time. The OKCIC staff uses this information to create fun and effective nutrition-and physical activity-based activities that re-enforce the lifestyle modifications necessary to maintain a healthy weight and reduce the risk for Type 2 diabetes. Each disease prevention experience includes a nutrition and physical activity component.

Ms. Sunday-Allen reports that outcomes after post-programming demonstrate that the "patient population experienced a substantial decrease in BMI percentile, the pediatric gauge for weight. In fact, the average BMI percentile dipped less than the level used for overweight classification (80th percentile), which is an encouraging sign of positive disease prevention progress. The change in BMI percentile may be a result of the significant decrease in sugar-sweetened beverage consumption and a decrease in sedentary screen time usage. While time in physical activity did decrease, the average remains above the Center for Disease Control's recommendation. These programs are made possible by SDPI funds for health educators, which include registered dietitians, physical activity specialists and support personnel as well as for venue rental, program supplies, and food."

Ms. Sunday-Allen recognizes that OKCIC's significant anti-diabetes effort would not have been possible without SDPI funds, and she strongly urges the Congress to reauthorize the program before the end of the fiscal year.

Let's finish our survey of how specific UIHPs are using SDPI funds by heading to the west coast. First, let's hear from the *Native American Rehabilitation Association of the Northwest (NARA)*, which serves eight locations in the Greater Portland Area. NARA focuses its diabetes efforts on screening, prevention, early diagnosis, and mitigating against complications caused by diabetes. Using SDPI funds since 1999, NARA has established a stable, cohesive, multi-disciplinary clinical group with more than 65 years of combined experience that serves over 500 people with diabetes and 1,000 patients with prediabetes.

NARA celebrated the success of its diabetes prevention program in 2016, receiving plaudits from lawmakers and public health experts alike. Since NARA first offered prevention classes in June 2006, the 133 graduates who completed the 20-week lifestyle balance curriculum—which includes weekly group meetings, tracking food intake, and increasing physical activity—collectively lost 1,350 pounds and 213 inches from their waist. NARA reports that prevention program graduates eat less unhealthy food, and more fruits, vegetables, and whole grains. NARA staff continue to meet with graduates monthly and support them as they strive to change their lifestyles.

NARA sees cultural competency and community partnerships as keys to its success in its fight against diabetes, striving to achieve a visible presence at community gatherings, cultural activities and powwows, in order to provide diabetes education and outreach.

NARA partners with the Casey Eye Institute's Outreach Team at Oregon Health Sciences University, which uses the team's mobile eye van to provide free dilated eye exams and prescriptions for glasses twice a year to the program's patients with diabetes. NARA also partners with the Mount Tabor podiatry office, which often treats the program's uninsured patients free of charge.

NARA shares best practices with the Northwest Portland Area Indian Health Board and local tribal organizations as well as the American Diabetes Association.

And through a partnership with mental and behavioral consultants, almost forty patients with poorly controlled diabetes (i.e., A1C greater than 9.0 percent) have been screened using a culturally-specific trauma examination process. The results indicate a strong correlation between a history of personal, past and/or intergenerational trauma and poorly-controlled diabetes. When patients screen positive for trauma, the behavioral health consultant coordinates referrals to a mental health consultant.

NARA successfully uses Saturday diabetes clinics, which are the program's convenient "one-stop-shop" clinic for people with diabetes to receive their annual diabetes "tune-up." Services provided at these clinics are podiatry, nutrition and exercise counseling, foot and nail care education, immunizations, laboratory testing, medication adjustments, diabetes education, and digital retinal screening. In fact, the percentages of patients completing a foot exam (97 percent vs 80 percent), eye exam

(78 percent vs 51 percent) and diabetes education (96 percent vs 84 percent) were higher for Saturday diabetes clinic participants than the general NARA diabetes patient population.

If the Congress fails to reauthorize SDPI, NARA would no longer be able to provide the Portland Indian community with the following services: diabetes screening; diabetes prevention; diabetes self-management education classes; nutrition and exercise counseling, podiatry services, retinal imaging services, and dilated eye exams for diabetics; and case-management for patients with prediabetes and diabetes.

Now, let's head south to California, where the *Indian Health Center of Santa Clara Valley (IHCSCV)* has established a holistic anti-diabetes program for education, prevention, and treatment that is an example for the general population of northern California.

IHCSCV's education effort is led by a registered nurse and it is further staffed with health educators, who provide one-on-one and group education about diabetes, teaching patients how to prevent the onset of the disease and mitigate against its complications—whether at the patient's home, at the program's wellness center, or at other health care facilities. Almost one-third of the budget for the wellness center has been paid for by SDPI funds.

IHCSCV's diabetes program, which was originally funded by SDPI, works to prevent or delay the onset of diabetes through manageable lifestyle changes. Although the SDPI grant expired last year, IHCSCV continues its fight against diabetes because of its continued harshly disproportionate impact on the Indian community in Northern California.

IHCSCV's primary care staff at the main facility as well as at three family practice clinics, and one pediatric clinic used SDPI funds to provide patients with the tools they need to manage their condition, including glucometers, test strips, lancets, blood sugar logs, pill cutters, diabetes socks, feet mirrors, and oral health supplies. Patients whose condition is more problematic benefit from intensive case-management.

IHCSCV's anti-diabetes effort is impressive in its comprehensiveness. IHCSCV has a fitness center that is free for all patients and available to patients at all skill levels. Many fitness classes are designed for patients who are elderly or have limited mobility, including Zumba and chair exercise classes. IHCSCV's fitness coordinator is also a personal trainer, who is able to offer one-on-one personal training to patients of all ages and skill levels.

IHCSCV helps its diabetes patients overcome transportation barriers imposed by limited mobility and social isolation. The program provides transportation for medical, dental, counseling, and specialty appointments, as well as to the wellness center and community events that are hosted for the Indian community by IHCSCV and its partners.

IHCSCV's diabetes patients often have many health complications and are facing other obstacles to their health—including homelessness, mental disabilities, limited income, and lack of health insurance. IHCSCV's case management team works closely with the patients and their primary care providers to coordinate the care within and outside of the program. The case management team arranges appointments with dentists, licensed clinical social workers, and psychiatrists at the program as well as with outside specialists like cardiologists, endocrinologists, nephrologists, and oncologists. In fact, some IHCSCV managers speak with their patients almost daily.

Like other UIHPs, IHCSCV believes it is imperative to reauthorize SDPI. Despite its accomplishments in the fight against diabetes, the program continues to treat new Indian patients with diabetes. Loss of SDPI funds would result in a significant decrease in access to transportation, which could mean that many patients would be less likely to receive the regular care necessary to control their diabetes. Loss of SDPI funds would also prevent IHCSCV from engaging in its aggressive, comprehensive case management or providing diabetes refreshers, which are two hour education classes specifically tailored for Indian patients with diabetes.

Finally, let's head north, to the Seattle Indian Health Board (SIHB). Thanks to the SDPI funds, they have a diabetic team that provides a comprehensive case management team consisting of a nutritionist, RN, MA, case manager, and PharmD. This team has been able to provide robust case management services that supplement the care our patients receive from their primary care provider.

The services they provide because of the SDPI program include diabetes and lifestyle education, assistance developing and reaching self-care goals, support for well-being, referral assistance, etc. The program has also provided group education classes on topics including exercise, diet, and general diabetes education. SDPI funding has also provided onsite optometry and podiatry specialty services for our diabetic patients.

Without SDPI, SIHB would anticipate at least a 75 percent reduction in the diabetic case management services that they currently provide. They would also lose the ability to track and follow up with diabetic patients who were lost from care or have poor follow-up. This would inevitably lead to poorer outcomes for the patients and increased medical costs for the entire health system.

NCUIH appreciates the opportunity to testify about the challenging but promising work of UIHPs in educating against, preventing, and treating diabetes which have, literally, saved and transformed lives in Indian Country. So much of that work would not have been possible without SDPI, which is why NCUIH strongly urges the Committee to ensure that the program continues without any interruption. Quite simply, SDPI must be reauthorized if Indian Country is to educate against, treat, and prevent the terrible scourge that is diabetes. Thank you for your consideration. Please contact NCUIH if you have any questions about our testimony.

*Here is an appreciative note Ms. Keeler received from one SDUIH patient about the program's SDPI-funded diabetes treatment:

"I just wanted to touch base with you and thank you for getting me involved in the program. If you ever had any doubts about the importance of it, I want to let you know I did go to my eye exam and they did find I had cataracts due to my diabetes. So this program, in the long run will have saved my life. I just wanted to let you know what they found. This has certainly, with no pun intended, opened my eyes to my responsibility in regards to my diabetes. Again-just a call to say thank you. Also, my children both have pre-diabetes and would like them to start coming to your facility. But anyway, this work is so important and thank you again!"

*Sally is a 12-year-old participant in IHCRC's Running Strong youth run club. A wonderful but unexpected outcome of the club is that many parents are inspired to participate with their children, and Sally's mother registered to run alongside her daughter in a 5K.

"I did my first 5K!!! I was not in the front of the pack but I wasn't the last one either so I will take that as a win!!! I did it for my amazing daughter Sally who of course kicked my butt. She did great in her first 5K also. I am so proud. Wished I could have seen her come over the finish line. I did meet some very sweet ladies that helped me along the way. And a huge thanks to Sally's run club!!! You all are rock stars."

One week later, there was another 5K—this one in brutally cold weather. Sally's mom commented:

"Today I finished another 5K with the help of my amazing daughter. She ran back and got me and helped me finish strong. She is such an amazing kid. Although the running is hard I love that we are doing it together. Even if she kicks my butt (lol). It is something we can enjoy and push each other with. All of it wouldn't be possible without her amazing run group and coach Jennie Howard. We could never thank you enough."

*Here is the success story of one family in which every member weighed in excess of 250 pounds when they began IHCRC's program:

"I wanted to let you know what a positive move this has been for our whole family. The first positive is our weight loss. Our oldest son lost 109 pounds during the past year. His younger brother only lost 17 pounds but his grades increased as his weight has decreased. I can't thank you enough for the changes that you have brought to my family! I just can't believe the positive outcome of exercise!

"We have stopped drinking sweet tea and we haven't eliminated sweets but we only have them on special occasions. We have also tried to limit our bread/other sugar intake. A big deal for us was portion size, we seen nothing wrong with eating 2 or 3 plates. Now we try to only have 1. We work out at least 5 times a week. We try to go 7 days a week but sometimes other activities interfere (work/school). We also play volleyball and basketball.

"We are a healthy family and working towards improving that even more and we enjoy it!!! I began using my Facebook page as an exercise log to help keep me accountable. This in turn has encouraged many of my friends to begin walking or working out. I am motivating others and it feels awesome! I have people private message me about what they are trying to do because they don't want to go public in case they fail, and I encourage them that a little exercise is better than none and there is no failing when you are doing something to move your body around.

"My husband was diagnosed borderline diabetic. Diabetes runs on his side of the family and he has seen all the struggles his dad has before he passed away from it. We are hoping that all of the things we have done will defeat that disease and break the cycle."

*Here are five testimonials from patients who have been treated for diabetes by OKCIC.

1. GS, a proud "great great grandpa" and an OKCIC patient for more than 30 years, states:

"Different foot doctors all wanted to cut off my foot. I would take off my shoes and show them my foot and they all said if they didn't take off my foot, they'd have to take off my leg up my knee". I came to Oklahoma City Indian Clinic and saw the Wound Care Team. They said, 'We can save that!' Everyone was so positive here. OKCIC gave me support care, the podiatrist and other doctors have been a great help."

2. "Six years ago I was approached by a member of the Steps to Achieve Results (STAR) program in the Oklahoma City Indian Clinic wellness center. I was told about an upcoming Diabetes Alert Day.I was given an appointment with my provider and I found out I was pre-diabetic. I have seen diabetes at its worst. So, of course when I learned I was pre-diabetic, I wanted to learn as much as I could in order to keep from becoming diabetic. I did not want my children to see me like I saw my dad. I knew they would take care of me, but I did not want them to have to. I enrolled in the STAR program where I learned how to count my daily fat grams and calories. I also learned how to prepare my food differently. I learned how to lose 7 percent of my starting weight and how to keep it off by adding activity with my food choices. I learned a lot and after 16 weeks finished the program. After being in the program, I thought it would be interesting to work in the medical field helping my Native people. In time, an opportunity arose and a life coach position became available. I applied and now am a proud member of the STAR team for a little over 4 and half years. In the process, I have also obtained a certified personal trainer certificate. I get to help my Native brothers and sisters in a rewarding capacity by using my experience and the strength of the curriculum. Through the many acquaintances, I have made some lifelong friendships."

3. "I have lost a total of 15 pounds with the Star program. I have increased my activity and I feel amazing as the result. I feel I'm not out of breathe anymore when doing cardio. I am an active runner and with all the pounds being taken away my legs don't hurt like they use to when running last spring. I have also seen results as my pull ups are looking a lot better than they ever have because I am down 15 pounds from what I had started with. The benefits are incredible. I get compliments from so many people wondering what I am doing. This program does not make me feel like it is a diet but a true lifestyle change. This class has truly helped me with my diet completely. This class has helped me learn about proteins and I don't have to get it from chicken. My recipes and lunches have been so much more creative because of this class and I am so thankful it has brought me to this place of being healthy and happy. I love how the program is setup because it's in baby steps and the staff has been amazing because when I would slip, they got me back on track so now it's just a habit to stay on the healthy lifestyle."

4. "STAR cooking and Get SET has helped me out a lot. It has motivated me to come into the clinic and exercise. STAR cooking has taught me how to cook properly for my health and to stay on the right diet plan to continue my health management. The reason I come to STAR cooking is because I have high blood pressure, which caused my kidneys to fail. The diet plan for diabetics is similar for what I need to do on my diet plan with my health issues. I'm a 74-year-old woman and this helps me to keep healthy."

5. BL has managed to lose 20 pounds since she began the STAR program. By the end of the initial 8 weeks, she managed to lose 12 pounds:

"Prior to my participation in the STAR Program I felt that I would be unable to make significant changes to my weight and to my overall health. I have tried other methods and programs that were not effective. The life coaches celebrated even the smallest improvements and gave me different options to overcome obstacles as well. The STAR program has equipped me with tools and resources so that I can make informed changes that will result in a healthier future."

○